D0059504

FOOD

The centrality of food in life, and the importance of food as life, is undeniable. As a source of biological substrates, personal pleasure and political power, food is and has been an enduring requirement of human biological, social and cultural existence. In recent years, interest in food has increased across the academic, public and popular spheres, fuelled by popular media's constant play on the role of food and body size, and food and cooking, as a mass spectacle for TV audiences.

In *Food*, John Coveney examines 'food as …' humanness, identity, politics, industry, regulation, the environment and justice. He explores how food helps us understand what it means to be human. Through food, we construct our social identities, our families and communities. But this Shortcut also highlights the tensions between the industrialisation of food, the environment and the fair (or otherwise) worldwide distribution of food. It considers how the food industries, on which most of us have to rely, have also had direct effects on our bodies – whether through diet and longevity, or the development of illness and disease.

This book is for students and general readers alike – for anyone with a fascination with food. It questions the idea that food is merely something inert on the plate. Instead, it shows how influential, symbolic, powerful and transformative food has come to be.

John Coveney is a Professor of Public Health at Flinders University, Adelaide, South Australia. He is the author of, among other works, *Food, Morals and Meaning* (2nd edition, Routledge).

SHORTCUTS – "Little Books on Big Issues"

Series Editor: Anthony Elliott is Director of the Hawke Research Institute, where he is Research Professor of Sociology at the University of South Australia.

Shortcuts is a major new series of concise, accessible introductions to some of the major issues of our times. The series is developed as an A to Z coverage of emergent or new social, cultural and political phenomena. Issues and topics covered range from food to fat, from climate change to suicide bombing, from love to zombies. Whilst the principal focus of *Shortcuts* is the relevance of current issues, topics and debates to the social sciences and humanities, the books should also appeal to a wider audience seeking guidance on how to engage with today's leading social, political and philosophical debates.

Titles in the series:

Confronting Climate Change
Constance Lever-Tracy

Planet Sport
Kath Woodward

Feelings
Stephen Frosh

Fat
Deborah Lupton

Suicide Bombings
Riaz Hassan

Reinvention
Anthony Elliott

Web 2.0
Sam Han

Panic
Keith Tester

Global Finance
Robert J. Holton

Love
Tom Inglis

Freedom
Nick Stevenson

Food
John Coveney

Food

John Coveney

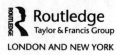

Routledge
Taylor & Francis Group

LONDON AND NEW YORK

First published 2014
by Routledge
2 Park Square, Milton Park, Abingdon, Oxon OX14 4RN

Simultaneously published in the USA and Canada
by Routledge
711 Third Avenue, New York, NY 10017

*Routledge is an imprint of the Taylor & Francis Group, an informa
business*

© 2014 John Coveney

The right of John Coveney to be identified as author of this work
has been asserted by him in accordance with sections 77 and 78 of
the Copyright, Designs and Patents Act 1988.

All rights reserved. No part of this book may be reprinted or
reproduced or utilised in any form or by any electronic,
mechanical, or other means, now known or hereafter invented,
including photocopying and recording, or in any information
storage or retrieval system, without permission in writing from the
publishers.

Trademark notice: Product or corporate names may be trademarks or
registered trademarks, and are used only for identification and
explanation without intent to infringe.

British Library Cataloguing in Publication Data
A catalogue record for this book is available from the British
Library

Library of Congress Cataloging-in-Publication Data
Coveney, John.
Food/John Coveney.
pages cm. -- (Shortcuts)
Includes bibliographical references and index.
1. Food--Social aspects. 2. Food in popular culture. 3. Food
habits. 4. Food preferences. I. Title.
TX357.C585 2013
641.3--dc23
2012051054

ISBN: 978-0-415-52445-2 (hbk)
ISBN: 978-0-415-52446-9 (pbk)
ISBN: 978-0-203-51988-2 (ebk)

Typeset in Bembo
by Taylor & Francis Books

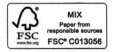

Printed and bound in Great Britain by
TJ International Ltd, Padstow, Cornwall

For Jean, Joan and Michael

Contents

Series editor's foreword   viii
Acknowledgements   ix

Introduction   1

1   Food as ... humanness   6

2   Food as ... identity   19

3   Food as ... politics   32

4   Food as ... industry   45

5   Food as ... regulation   60

6   Food as ... the environment   73

7   Food as ... justice   87

References   100
Index   101

SERIES EDITOR'S FOREWORD

Shortcuts is a major new series of concise, accessible introductions to some of the major issues of our times. The series is developed as an A to Z coverage of emergent or new social, cultural and political phenomena. Issues and topics covered range from finance to fat, from climate change to zombies, from love to suicide bombing. Whilst the principal focus of *Shortcuts* is the relevance of current issues, topics and debates to the social sciences and humanities, the books should also appeal to a wider audience seeking guidance on how to engage with today's leading social, political and philosophical debates.

Written with penetrating insight and admirable clarity, John Coveney's contribution to *Shortcuts* situates food in its wider social, economic, political and environmental contexts. Against the backdrop of industrial capitalism, Coveney is out to demonstrate that food is a phenomenon that bridges the biological and symbolic, the erotic and ethical, the affective and rational, at the level of everyday life. Significantly, Coveney also deftly reveals that food, in our own time, has come to mean lifestyle, diet, fashion, marketing, advertising and global political governance. *Food* is a provocative Shortcut on one of the most basic – but most pressing – issues of our time.

Anthony Elliott

Acknowledgements

Many thanks to my colleagues and co-workers who make food research, teaching and broadcasting so satisfying and rewarding.

INTRODUCTION

I have a friend who is obsessed by food. His interests go far beyond merely cooking and eating. The very idea of food engages him; food and history, food and culture, food and economics. He knows it all. It has to be said that having a discussion with my friend, let's call him Fred – Fred the Foodie – can be a trial. Inevitably he steers every subject around to a food theme. A question about whether he has seen a recent film will inevitably lead to a discussion about the movie's food scene or food-related event, however minor or incidental. A mention of politics will trigger an outpouring about the political impact on food's availability, affordability and accessibility. Of course, the consequences of talking about travel with Fred are obvious – a discussion about the local food delicacies and delights. Fred's favourite popular music is anything sung by the Beatles, mostly because mentions of food and drink crop up so often in their songs.

I have to say that I have on occasions found Fred the Foodie somewhat trying. How anyone could hold and sustain an interest so profound in food was, to be honest, beyond me. However, during the writing of this book I began to think of Fred rather differently. I could see that beyond providing us with the obvious pleasures of eating and drinking, food plays a central role in virtually all aspects of our lives. From providing us with sustenance, to lubricating social engagements, to enriching our cultural practices, to creating big business, to destroying local economies and endangering lifestyles, food is it.

I began to see that the central role of food is best understood by reformulating our perception of it. I now think about food entirely differently. I now understand how it fits into our biological, social, cultural, historical and economic development. I realise that food is never just an object on a plate or a menu. Food always does something more than just being there. It nurtures. It speaks. It travels. It calculates. It identifies. It joins. It separates. It demarcates. It historicises. It symbolises. It empowers. It disempowers.

So profound is our relationship with food that I now find it easy to say that food is, indeed, who we are. This is true literally, because our material bodies are made up of components that were once food. It is also true metaphorically, because food has been, and still is, an identifier and maker of class, culture and civilisation.

However, one of the things that struck me about my new appreciation of food – and, indeed, of Fred – is that, starting about 100 years ago, and more rapidly in the last 30 years, we have let go of food. We have outsourced it to others who are largely invisible and unknown to us. The thought of this frightens and shocks me. This is because in abrogating our relationship with food we have, I believe, cut ourselves free of the very substance that makes us and joins us.

In this 'Shortcuts' book I want to show the making and joining that food does. I want to illustrate how, using food as a lens, we can know, understand and appreciate a number of matters, concerns and developments that are germane to biological, social and political discourse today. Food also allows us to appreciate our history, and that of others.

Thus the purpose of this book is to show how by refracting a number of issues through a food lens, we can better understand many aspects of human development. I hope, like me, you will be transformed by thinking about food as a doing thing, rather than merely a being thing.

By virtue of being a 'Shortcut' to food, the contents of this book have been deliberately kept pithy and succinct. Nevertheless, it roams over the main food issues facing us today, looking at different facets and interconnections. Thus the book has seven chapters, each of which talks about food as something. So the first chapter looks at food as humanness. The focus here is on how food has shaped human growth and development. These terms, human growth and development, crop up a lot in this book, so some explanation is needed here. In this book human development is taken to mean the ways in which we have developed biologically, socially and culturally. Of course, we can see human development as biology in action when we watch children get bigger and taller. The role of food in this change is fundamental, and something we take for granted. And stopping for a moment to consider how miraculous this change is truly humbles me. But equally humbling is the way in which food has been at the centre of social and cultural transformations. For centuries, and indeed, still today, food has been the major factor in lives of individuals, groups and communities. There is even one story, yet to be validated, that it was during the first use of fire and the cooking of meat that *Homo sapiens* began communicating, cooperating and socialising. In other words, our early commensality – literally sharing the table – was the key to human connectedness and sociality. Indeed, the core traits that make us human. Chapter 1 looks at the ways in which food is at the centre of medieval and modern human sciences. And through food we understand what it means to be human.

Chapter 2 develops this theme more by looking at food as identity. The argument here is that food elements build us biologically – so back to human development. We look also at the ways in which food is used to construct social identities. That is to say, the ways in which we use food as a class divider and cultural glue. Chapter 3 explores food as politics. This does not mean politics as in 'government' (which comes in Chapter 4). In this context politics concerns the ways that we live together in certain arrangements – like families and communities – and the rules that are used to organise those arrangements. Food in families is a political topic from many angles. For example, the work undertaken in making food into dishes and meals is usually completed by women, and this has a politics of its own that we explore. Similarly, community movements are increasingly organising themselves around food, and food-based movements are some of the most vocal and influential movements in bringing about change. Chapter 4 concerns food as regulation. Regulation here is defined as that which gives us access (or not) to food. In this chapter we explore regulation in the form of law and legislation. But we also look at self-regulation and the ways in which other forms of authority are used to control our eating. In Chapter 5 we look at food as industry. By any measure the industrialisation of food is a remarkable achievement, and in the eyes of many a stand-out success story in human development. Being able to control food supply in a way that our ancestors would not have dreamed of is incredible. Stand in any supermarket and marvel at the range and quality of food available. And the price. However, there is a downside to this, and the idea of *Big Food* is discussed in terms of its formation and its consequences. Chapter 6 looks at food as environment, noting that food production has, for thousands of years, had an uneasy relationship with the environment, in some cases causing the devastation of arable land into what are now deserts. The destruction of the soil and the depletion of fish stocks are all a consequence of food production. More recently, the focus on climate change has implicated food production in the generation of the greenhouse gases that are thought to be responsible for extreme weather events which are experienced across the world. Finally, Chapter 7, food as justice, looks at the ways in which some people get to eat and others do not. This chapter does not only look at the injustices concerned with who gets what quantity of food; it also looks at who gets what in terms of food quality, noting that the introduction of foods to less well-off countries has undermined local food cultures and food production knowledge.

The seven chapters all have one thing in common: they each question the idea that food is merely something inert on the plate. Instead, food is seen to be influential, symbolic, powerful and transformative. Fred the Foodie would be very pleased with this book.

1

FOOD AS ... HUMANNESS

Introduction

In this chapter we will look at the fundamental role played by food in human development. We will look at how food was central to early medicine as a correction, not only to repair physical health but also to restore moral character. This role of food is largely overlooked today, because the medieval science in which it belongs faded in history. But this did not diminish the centrality of food in human development and understanding. For as the human science differentiated into what we now understand as biology, psychology, sociology, anthropology and so on, food continued to play a central role in pursuits to understand what it means to be 'human'. In this central role food is, of course, never merely things on a plate. Indeed, the central foundation of this book is that food is never just 'food', but is always symbolic of other capabilities and capacities, depending on the lens used.

It goes without saying that we regard food as a necessity for life. We see that all living things need some kind of food, and indeed water, in order to continue living. Food constitutes us and sustains us. Our knowledge of food and of the elements in food, the basic building blocks of food, allow us to know how, at every level of life, food plays an essential role in keeping us going. From the cellular angle we know that various nutrients are essential for the reproduction of new cells for the body. From the organ level we know that a variety of food elements are needed for proper growth and maintenance. And from a systems level we know that food is needed to regulate particular pathways. We acknowledge the discoveries in molecular biology, anatomy, physiology and biochemistry for these understandings. Of course, as we will see in later chapters, we also acknowledge the science of nutrition itself for helping build into the discoveries of physiological and biochemical systems our knowledge of nutrients.

There is, however, another science, more like an art, much older than the ones already mentioned, which deserves some credit for laying the foundations for how we understand the role of food and the body in health and illness. The field is *dietetics*, and it has a long and interesting history.

The dietetics

Today we often collapse together the knowledge of nutrition and dietetics. A distinction could be made, however, that nutrition is about the science of food and dietetics is about applying that science to address illness. So people are often required to see a dietitian if they have a medical condition in which food plays a role to help manage it. Later, in Chapter 6, we will touch on the fact that dietetics in ancient Greece was much more than this therapeutic role. It concerned the management of everyday life (*diete* meaning daily regime). In this chapter, however, we will look at the way in which food has long been considered essential, not only for addressing physical health, but also for correcting one's psychological wellbeing, and indeed one's character and temperament. This role played by food has a long history in western culture, and indeed in other cultures (although we will not be able to look closely beyond our own). To a large extent these properties of food were foundational to the development of food cultures and gastronomies. Thus many of the differences we see now in food cultures – and indeed celebrate, with an appreciation of, say, French, Italian, and other cuisines – will have been influenced by early thinking about food and its central role in creating and sustaining life at all levels. To better understand this early thinking we need to look at how food linked with early ideas of medicine in western history.

Food, body and soul

For more than 1,000 years in western culture, and longer in some others, a system of understanding the mind and the body reigned supreme. It was based on a set of principles that are traceable to early Greece – and indeed to Hippocrates, who is considered to be the father of medicine. The system was refined by Galen of Pergamum (AD 129–216?), whose writings on the subject were copious. The system was based on a belief that the body relied on four fluids, or humors, that circulated throughout the system. The fluids had independent properties, but they also had a relationship with each other, so careful balance of the humors was required. The humoral fluids were blood, yellow bile (or choler), black bile, and phlegm. Each of these was credited with having different and distinctive effects on the body, making it more or less vulnerable to various sicknesses. Having too little or too much of one humor could create a susceptibility to particular diseases.

Moreover, once illness struck, the re-balancing of the humors was necessary to fight the problem and return the individual to wellness. However, to think of the humors as almost drugs for the body is to miss a number of other important functions they played. For, while humors were of obvious importance to physiological functioning, they were also vital for psychological, and indeed moral, fitness. Because each humor was endowed with particular strengths and weaknesses, humoral balance was thought to influence a person's temperament, character and mood. This was because each humor had a particular set of characteristics. Blood is considered hot and moist; choler is hot and dry; black bile is cold and dry; and phlegm is cold and moist. The mixing together of the humors provided an individual's overall disposition. For example, blood was associated with being sanguine – that is, healthy and merry; choler bestowed the property of quickness of wit but also quickness of anger; black bile brought melancholy, a sad and solitary disposition; and phlegm provided a calm, cool, detached, even bland nature.

Food and the humors

There were many things that could influence the humors. Certain physiological states could have an effect – for example, a woman's menstrual cycle, or a person's age. Also, as we have mentioned, pathological states could influence humors. However, the humors could also be influenced by external forces, such as the time of year, geography and even the cosmos, since astrological arrangements and alignments could influence one's humoral balance. Thus humoral medicine linked individuals to their social, geographical and indeed cosmological environments.

Importantly, it was through food and drink that the humors were corrected and re-balanced, and complexion, or personal nature, restored. (Incidentally, it was believed that the humoral state of an individual could be read from their skin, thus the term 'complexion' became synonymous with skin tone and colour.)

It was thus the role of dietetics to recommend what to eat and drink not only when people were physically ill, but also when they felt psychologically indisposed or weak of character. This was because one's mood and disposition was influenced by humoral balance. And because of the natural flux of one's psycho-somatic wellbeing, as well as the changing terrestrial and extra-terrestrial elements, there was a constant need to pay attention to diet to re-adjust and re-calibrate body and mind. Attention to diet was also necessary because foods could enhance certain humoral effects. For example, black pepper was choler-producing, and the use of black pepper in the diet provided dietitians with at least two possibilities: recommend more of it when a more choleric effect was required (such as to combat an overly sanguine disposition), or less of it when an individual's complexion was regarded to be imbalanced towards yellow bile.

The point is to emphasise the centrality of food and drink to the person themselves: their physiology, psychology, pathology, character, mood and moral dispositions. In other words, food was *life*, in every aspect of the meaning – food was humanness. While the humoral theory has roots in ancient Greece and Rome, this model of thinking exploded during the early Renaissance. According to Ken Albala (in his book *Eating Right in the Renaissance*), this was for a number of reasons, not least of which was the outpouring of medical texts and treatises made possible by the growth of the printing and bookbinding industries. These technologies made available large archives concerned with maladies and medicine. And because humoral theory was central to medicine, writings on the humors were plentiful. However, another reason for the high volume of books on the subject was the changing nature of thinking about moral and ethical comportment. That is to say, the way people thought about themselves as 'selves' was transformed.

The work of Michel Foucault (in *The Order of Things*) provides us with a description of this transformation of individual subjectivity during and after the Renaissance, where attention paid to what might be described as the 'interiority of self' changed. Essentially a new awareness of, and thinking about, what it meant to be a person. Foucault called this new person, or subject, the 'empirico-transcendental doublet' to register the way in which an individual's everyday experiences are matched with moral imperatives; that is, what one was required to do. The transformation from a medieval human understanding of government or control to a different form of authority that had a greater focus on self-control was swift and powerful. Thus an audience was ripe for works and manuals on how to be a better subject – in every aspect of personal and civil life. Of course, religion and religious texts had long provided sources of inspiration for enhancing one's moral character. However, the body's humoral system, and methods to adjust it, provided a ready and secular course of action outside the church on ways of leading a better, more enhanced way of living. And dietetics played a central role in the management of living through the ability of food to directly interact with the humoral elements.

This highly interactive system could not be more different from that which we understand today, where we regard our 'selves' as sentient, conscious minds complete with exterior bodies. Although there is recognition that our psychology does interact with our physiology – to use a fairly shallow example, when we mentally experience shame or guilt, we often physically blush – the mind and body are regarded as separated. In humoral theory, however, the mind and body were intimately linked, and were under the influence of external elements such as food and drink, as well as time, place and astrological pattern. The role of the diet in medicine was therefore paramount.

Another chief consideration was that diets were highly individualised, not only because of disposition, but also because of individual situations and experiences. Thus uniform, broad recommendations were rare. However, there were general guidelines, mostly about the value of particular foods. For example, melons and cucumbers were to be avoided, being thought to contain only water, which could get trapped and render the food indigestible, leading to putrefaction within the body. Fruits were also regarded with suspicion for similar reasons. While differing in detail, the humoral theory was widespread across Europe, with a heyday, as noted earlier, during the European Renaissance. A similar system of thought was present in the Arabic world.

In thinking about this we should acknowledge that the dietetics as explained so far was not available to all – mostly only to those who could afford to consider choices in what they ate and drank. Essentially, this meant people of affluence. Also, we must not think that dietaries were followed to the letter. Then, as now, there were authorities that spoke on what the ideal would be, generally and individually, but the extent to which these prescriptions and recommendations were followed is unknown. What we do know is that dietetics as expressed in the humoral theory of medicine had unifying influence about what is good to eat and drink, albeit individualised according to personal requirements. As the popularity for humoral explanations of what is good to eat faded, they were replaced by other forms of knowledge.

There is much debate about whether the dietetics informed or was informed by culinary practices. Indeed, food historian Barbara Santich shows how the basis for the humors, which emphasised good food, is foundational to gastronomy. Both humoral medicine and gastronomy seek to exercise discrimination and judgement about what is prudent and good to eat, not only as sustenance, but also as a route to better living and well-being. This understanding of gastronomy is far from that which sees it as a preoccupation with fine, rich or elaborated foods and dishes. The dietetic–gastronomic understanding of diet sees food as *life*, in all manifestations. Food is not merely what arrives on a plate, nor is it only what is prepared for the table. Food is the essence of life, even the spirit of living.

What is good to eat?

Social nutritionist Pat Crotty is famous for saying that the mouth divides our understanding of food. She describes this separation as the 'pre-swallowing' and 'post-swallowing' cultures. By this she means that food is understood today both from the viewpoint of psycho-social-cultural perspectives (pre-swallowing) and from the perspective of knowledge of food through nutrient interactions with bodily systems (post-swallowing). Of course, no such distinctions were possible under the earlier humoral theories of dietetics, where pre- and post-swallowing knowledges were intimately linked. However, within contemporary understandings and distinctions it is possible to separate out how individual disciplines and fields of knowledge draw on food and indeed food choice to explain aspects of our very 'humanness' in all the various manifestations.

How do we understand food choice?

According to some researchers, food choice is clearly something that can be understood solely in terms of biology and psychology. Within this understanding the selection of foods can be separated into two distinct lines of inquiry. The first seeks to locate mechanisms that govern food choice within a person's biological and genetic make-up. It attempts to uncover so-called 'innate' processes that are regulated through biological precursors and chemical messengers. The second line of inquiry is closer to the area of behavioural psychology, and looks at food choice as a product of cognitive processes and conditioning, which themselves respond to various biological stimuli.

The first line of inquiry encompasses work on the genetic determination of food choice, based on the observation that food preferences tend to run in families. For example, investigations have demonstrated that the sensitivity to, say, bitter tastes may be genetically transmitted and a greater similarity in preferences for certain foods has been found between identical twins than between fraternal twins. Since each of the twin pairs was sharing the same home environment, the similarities in food choice represent a genetically transmitted trait rather than socially determined habits. Studies into so-called intrinsic tendencies have looked at taste preferences of infants, especially infants' responses to different tastes like sweet, sour and bitter. Apparently, even within hours of birth neonates prefer sweet tastes. The usual explanation for such taste preferences is in terms of 'nutritional wisdom', in which an innate dislike for bitterness and a liking for sweetness is believed to guide infants towards safer, more nutritious foods (for example, breast milk) and protect against harmful substances that are usually bitter or sour tasting. Pause here to notice how food is used to provide evidence for so-called innate traits or human tendencies. In other words, food preference in babies is used to describe our 'natural' humanness.

The notion of intrinsic or innate 'nutrition wisdom' was investigated in the late 1920s by Clara Davis. In an effort to see whether humans could instinctively choose the right kind of food, she conducted a longitudinal study with orphanage infants aged 6–9 months. Throughout the study the children were presented with a variety of foods and were allowed to select whateverthey wanted. Over a course of months the children tasted everything (including spoons, trays, paper). They apparently selected from a wide range of foods and grew and developed according to the norms of the day. Davis concluded that in infants there must be an innate mechanism which guides food choice in the direction of good nutrition. Davis' work became important to the theories about an innate basis of food choice in humans. The central tenet of these theories is that, given a free choice (that is, choice not constrained by 'culture'), humans are 'naturally' guided to nutritious diets. While Davis' conclusions have been criticised – mainly because the infants in her study were offered only wholesome foods and so could not help but construct healthy diets for themselves – the work is used as a starting point to understand so-called innate food choice mechanisms. This innateness takes as its starting point the biological make-up of humans: their physiological systems and their genetic precursors; properties that are considered to be predetermined and universal. Biology would assert that this is about the ways in which food, once ingested, breaks down to nutrients which form the building blocks of cells in every aspect of human growth, development, maintenance and repair. Indeed, it might be said that we are what we eat, biologically.

There is, however, debate about this claim by biology. Claude Fischler points out that biological adaptation often happens under the influence of cultural preference. We know, for example, that on a world scale most cultures do not consume milk after infancy; and in most cultures adults do not produce the enzyme, lactase, necessary to digest milk, lactose. In those cultures that choose to consume cows' milk, however, the human body has adapted and continues to produce lactase. The argument here is then that culture sometimes pre-determines biology, in this case through the production of lactase. This is a perfect example of the ways in which food provides a tangible insight into human development. By collapsing what are often separate understandings of what it means to be human – how did humans develop a particular biology? how does culture work so as to give specificity to human groups? – our dietary practices show how what we eat shapes life, at all levels.

Another example of how food shapes life is through the grounding of food choice in larger frameworks of human society and culture. As Gordon Tait points out, a number of psychological theories about eating disorders have been extended to include 'socio-cultural influences'. Good examples of these come from the writings of Susie Orbach, Naomi Wolf and Susan Bordo. Each author stresses that an understanding of eating problems in young women should be considered in terms of social structures in western culture, which both construct 'womanhood' and oppress women.

Studies of food have also been used to construct understandings of other oppressed groups. For example, the nineteenth-century social surveys by Charles Booth and Seebohm Rowntree on poverty in different parts of nineteenth-century England highlighted the problems of food for certain social groups. Indeed, Rowntree, in his work in northern England, not only highlighted poverty but also defined it by establishing a so-called 'poverty line'. This was based on how much people needed to earn to eat properly. Thus the very definition that marks 'poverty' was arrived at through understanding what and how much food is affordable. This is a perfect example of the centrality of food to understanding our social lives.

Sociologist Pierre Bourdieu, who has also studied the structure of social arrangements in regard to food choice, picks this up. In the survey described in *Distinctions: A Social Critique of the Judgement of Taste*, Bourdieu uses food and food choice to show how people are positioned in accordance with their class expectations – their collective consciousness – by virtue of what they eat. Thus, in a figurative and literal sense, we are (socially) what we eat, again showing that food is not merely something inert on our plate. It communicates meaning, purpose and structure to our social lives.

Finally, let us look at how anthropology has been interested in food as culture. According to anthropologist Anne Murcott, the study of food in human groups has been of central concern to anthropology almost since its inception. Perhaps the work of Claude Lévi-Strauss is the most significant and the most widely

quoted example of food and food choice. Working from supposed universal human activities, such as language and communication, Lévi-Strauss points to cooking as an event which is
undertaken by all known societies. And using methods borrowed
from structural linguistics, he attempts to show how cooking may
be understood as a fundamental human activity. Lévi-Strauss
believes that one of the primary binary oppositions that all
human cultures have to deal with is nature/culture relationship;
that is, humans are part of nature in that they are constituted as
biological beings, but humans are cultural in that they are socially
and culturally constituted too. Cooking thus represents an activity where humans transform nature into culture. The raw
is turned into the cooked. Nature can also transform food, but
this is done through rotting or fermenting. Out of these propo-
sitions Lévi-Strauss is able to construct a 'Culinary Triangle', the
points of which are represented by raw food, cooked food and
rotten food. Lévi-Strauss argues that cooking is a symbolic act; it
allows humans to communicate their 'humanness'. To cook food
and to rank food into the edible and the non-edible is, he
believes, a fundamental human trait. The propensity for this
action is a part of human nature; it is an integral structure within
the human mind.

Closing remarks about food as humanness

In this chapter we have looked at the ways in which food and
eating have been central to our understanding of a whole range
of disciplines in what might be regarded as the human sciences,
sciences that are about describing our humanness. Food is used to
illustrate how we are basically biological beings, with so-called
'innate' tendencies. Food is also used to demonstrate how we
construct our psychological and social worlds. It is not hard to
agree with Lévi-Strauss' assertion that food is fundamentally
linked to our humanness. Indeed, it would be hard to think of

any other human practice that plays such a central role to human development. This is not merely because we engage with food on a regular basis in order to survive, which while true, reduces food to a mere vehicle for nutrients and substrates for physiological functions. We use food to satisfy our psychological needs and we use food to construct our social and cultural lives. Returning to Lévi-Strauss, who believed that food is not so much good to eat as 'good to think', we can say that through food we understand ourselves and our 'selves'. Even though we do not use humoral theory to explain the role of food in our everyday lives, we continue to draw on food as a way of describing our humanness.

Further reading

Albala, K., *Eating Right in the Renaissance*. Berkeley, CA: University of California Press, 2002.

Bourdieu, P., *Distinction: A Social Critique of Taste*. London: Routledge & Kegan Paul, 1984.

Crotty, P., *Good Nutrition? Fact and Fashion in Dietary Advice*. St Leonards: Allen and Unwin, 1995.

Fischler, C., Food habits, social change and the nature/culture dilemma. *Social Science Information* 19, 937–53, 1980.

Foucault, M., *The Order of Things: An Archaeology of the Human Sciences*. Bristol: Tavistock, 1982.

Levi-Strauss, C. The Culinary Triangle. New Society, 22nd December, 937–940.

Santich, B., Menage à trois: gastronomy, health, medicine. *Journal of Gastronomy* 2 16–29, 1986.

Story, M. and Brown, J.E., Do children instinctively know what to eat? The studies of Clara Davis revisited. *New England Journal of Medicine* 316 (2), 103–6, 1987.

Tait, G., 'Anorexia Nevosa'; Ascetism, differentiation, government. *Australia and New Zealand Journal of Sociology* 29, 194–208, 1993.

2

FOOD AS ... IDENTITY

Introduction

In the previous chapter we looked at how food, over time, has defined what it means to be human. Moving from medieval medicine, where diet was central to constructing personality and character, to modern human sciences, we saw that food is in fact central to life, in its multiplicity of understandings. In other words, to say 'you are what you eat' is a biological truism, a social truth and a cultural axiom.

In this chapter we look further at the way in which food works to 'construct' us by virtue of its ability to create an identity for us, individually and collectively. We will start by looking at how food provides the basic building blocks that renew daily our bodies and thus influences our outer appearance, and what we show to the world. We will then look at how food provides a means of belonging to social and cultural groupings, again creating for us an identity. By way of giving us some direction we will draw again on Pat Crotty's distinction between pre-swallowing and post-swallowing understandings of food. That is to say, the way that we can understand the role of food in creating identity by looking at its effects on the body (post-swallowing). We can also see how food before it is eaten makes an identity for us.

How food makes us

We begin with the basics: that is, the acknowledgement that our bodies are, literally, renewed on a daily, weekly or monthly basis. Put simply, most of the cells that form the outside or the inside of my body were not there a month ago. Some cells were not there a week ago. All this is to say that the turnover of our body components happens both inwardly (our organs, our systems) and outwardly (our skin, our hair). Of course, also turning over and being renewed are the cells that make up the structure of the body, the muscles and the bones (and all the components).

It might seem obvious that this constant turning over of our bodies is happening; but not so obvious, perhaps, is why. We replenish cells for a number of reasons. For example, skin cells and hair that are being constantly lost need to be replaced, with new cells being formed and pushed to the surface (skin cell) or out of a follicle (hair). Thus the outward layer of our bodies – our exterior identity, so to speak – is constantly being eroded and new cells are needed to replace old. Without this process we would simply wear away.

Importantly, the inner surfaces of the body are also being replaced. For example, the lining of cells along our intestinal tract is dislodged every time we send food along. Most of these cells are broken down and reabsorbed further along the tract, but new ones have to take their place. Similarly, bone cells are turning over, albeit very slowly. This is because the building blocks of bones, such as calcium and phosphate, are often lost through elimination products like urine and faeces. In order to keep up the strength of bones, new cells have to be formed to replace those being lost. This is not the place for full-scale physiology, but suffice it to say that as cells are broken down and cellular components lost to the body, they need replacing. And to accomplish this replenishment three things are needed: food, water and air. The food component is the most complex of these three because diets comprise different foods and therefore different nutrients. And it is food nutrients that provide the 'bricks and mortar', and the necessary energy to fuel the replenishment processes.

Food makes us what we are

There are several implications that flow from the way food affects our outer identity. An obvious one is 'thinness' and 'fatness', each of which carries a particular identity through visual appearance. Another is 'youth' and 'ageing', which can be influenced by the food and diet we eat. All of these demonstrate that our actual 'look and feel', clearly part of our identity, are modified and modifiable by what food we eat. We will look at each of these in turn.

Thinness and fatness

The visual appearances that arise from too little or too much food are probably the most ancient ways in which food identity has been noticed. The wretchedness of too little food and the consequent visual appearance – sagging skin, visible bone structures, haggard, gaunt faces – have since early history been noticed as the outward appearance of poverty, scarcity and neediness. They convey the message that the sufferers of such an experience are in dire trouble and warrant assistance. Media images of requests for charity donations for those stricken by famine or food crises often comprise graphic depictions of extreme thinness, often with no description – because none is necessary. We get the message. We understand what has happened and what is needed. The identity of the images conveys immediately a need for food because the problem stems from failure to provide food.

However, thinness does not always provoke sympathy or a fast path to a cash donation. Another level or 'style' of thinness can provoke an entirely different image. When Wallace Simpson, the Duchess of Windsor, said 'a woman cannot be too rich or too thin', she was talking about how thinness plays out in certain social groups, where it conveys high social standing. Achieving that standing, thinness, requires adherence to a strict food regime that has an effect on the body to produce such a result. So here we see how food creates, by its effects on our physical exterior, another identity: one of power and high social status, instead of one displaying wretchedness and helplessness. In other words, food, by virtue of the work it does on the body, creates and conveys identity.

Of course, these identities are not universal, and do not have the same meaning in every culture. Thinness in some cultures in high social standing groups is regarded to be a disadvantage and does not communicate the same message of success as it does in other groups. A distinction can be made between European cultures and those in the Pacific region or parts of Africa, where larger bodies are made so through food and deliberate over-feeding. For example, the Annang community of Nigeria and communities in the Pacific islands of Tahiti and Nauru are reported to have fattening practices where brides-to-be are deliberately overfed to produce lusty and culturally attractive bodies. And, of course, Japanese Sumo wrestlers are on a strict diet of plenty to be able to perform adequately in the ring. These practices not only produce bodies with particular functions – fecundity and fertility for the brides-to-be and strength for the Sumos – but also bodies with the ability to convey messages about wealth and power.

We now turn to look more closely at fatness to examine how food works on the body to create and convey our exterior identity. This is an interesting example of the ways in which the identity created by fatness has changed historically. For a long time in western history, fatness, or corpulence, was prized. It expressed a sense of being able to afford enough food, not just to feed oneself, but also to overfeed oneself, and indeed one's family. Interestingly, diseases that were associated with over-feeding also carried high social cachet. For example, Porter and Rousseau show how in the eighteenth and nineteenth centuries, gout signified affluence in those it plagued. This was because gout was invariably only experienced by the wealthy, and was associated with consuming rich foods.

Fast-forward to the present, where overfeeding oneself and one's family is not the costly business it used to be. Far from it. In relation to household income, food prices have steadily fallen over the past 100 years; in the nineteenth century food costs comprised about 60 per cent or more of household expenditure, whereas today it has fallen to about 10 per cent for the average Australian family. In the US that figure is about 7 per cent. So overfeeding is not the sign of wealth that it once was, and a large body size created by excess food now conveys a totally different image. Research shows that fatness carries numerous stigmas for the individual. Ryan Stanley argues that overweight transgresses a number of social norms, such as moderation in eating, mindfulness of healthy bodies, and importantly a display of willpower or self-control. All of these attributes say something about the person. Thus, again, the ability of food to create and convey a particular identity is evident.

Food in the life cycle

All of this demonstrates the centrality of food in creating us. It also hints at another capacity of food: to nourish our growth, which, as a consequence of maturation, also provides us with

certain physical characteristics. In this area, one of the most illu-
minating roles that food can play is in the process of ageing. The
general process of ageing, including its mental features and the
physical outward appearance, is thought to be due to degenera-
tion through chain reactions that affect the body (caused by
so-called 'free radicals'). These reactions damage cells and accel-
erate their turnover and death. Some foods contain a range of
constituents which buffer the chain reactions, and eaten in the
right amounts are supposed to slow down the ageing effects.
Indeed, a number of authors, both popular and professional, have
written about ways in which, through food, the process of ageing
can be delayed. Some even hint at halting the ageing process
altogether, and, with the right diet, staying forever young.

Other reports suggest that a number of traditional diets – for
example, those eaten in parts of Japan and in the middle-European
country of Georgia – while not necessarily delaying the visible
effects of ageing, are able to ensure that people age productively
well into senior years. The general belief is that a varied and
well-balanced diet is able to support physical work, which leads
to a stronger, healthier body. Particular aspects of the diet have
been credited with conferring life-extending properties. So, for
example, diets high in seafood are believed to be responsible
for longevity in Osakans in Japan, and yoghurt and other fermented milk products have been thought to be some of the key
ingredients that extend the lives of Georgians.

Food, identity and self-identity

So far we have looked at how the post-swallowing role of food
creates for us specific identities, by virtue of its effects on our
shape, or morphology, or its effects on our ability to age or do
work, and creates for us an external identity that we show to the
world. We now look at the way in which food, even before it is
eaten, sends a powerful signal about who we are. That is to say,

the act of choosing, preparing and organising food has a role to play in communicating something about us to others.

The sociologist Pierre Bourdieu, who was mentioned in Chapter 1, has undertaken an extensive study of French social class. Unlike much work in this area that is interested in the ways in which access to material wealth creates conditions for life and labour, Bourdieu was also interested in the symbolic ways communicated by various living standards. His study roamed across numerous areas, including work, relationships and leisure activities. However, one aspect related to food, and he showed how food choice was a powerful signifier of class. Groups used food to communicate aspects of their wealth, and diet was a powerful vehicle of cultural and social identity. People interviewed spoke about belonging to certain groups on the basis of the food they chose to eat. So working-class groups were more inclined to choose and enjoy earthy food and they were more likely to see food as fuel for work. On the other hand, wealthier people talked about the aesthetics of food, the importance of the right food display, and the integration of food with the right kind of accoutrements, such as fine tableware and glassware.

Of course, it could be said that this display of wealth, through food, is nothing new; as we touched on earlier, the idea of a 'groaning table' as a symbol of someone's prosperity is a common phenomenon in many cultures. But Bourdieu found something different by showing that wealth did not actually mean a table full of food. Indeed, in 1960s France, for wealthier people the table could be modestly furnished and that was itself sufficient to communicate affluence. What mattered was quality, not quantity. These 'distinctions', as Bourdieu called them, were driven by what he called 'capitals', and 'cultural capital' was a powerful marker of identity, sending out to the world messages about who we are as social beings. But the communication of identity by food was not a one-way street – it did not just operate to send out the message. It also served to authorise for the individual an assurance about their social role. So eating vegetarian lasagne communicates to the individual a different message from eating a Big Mac. The first is perhaps a possible message to one's self-concern, even virtue, about individual health, and the health of the planet; the other communicates a connection and consistency with popular culture as a result of eating a globally recognised icon.

Food and health identity

This relationship between food and self is often overlooked in campaigns and initiatives that attempt to change people's eating habits to make them 'healthier'. This usually requires people eating more fruit and vegetables, more wholegrain cereals, low-fat products, etc. However, these changes are not merely changes in food choice, and not only require a change in the way we taste and appreciate food and flavour – itself something of a major achievement. It also requires a change in the way people see their selves and construct their own identities. 'Eating healthily' carries with it powerful signals about how we think and feel about our selves; these are often feelings of virtue and goodness which in some social groups are not the kinds of characteristics that sit comfortably with the things people want to communicate to others, as well as themselves. Similarly, eating 'unhealthily' for some people carries messages about a lack of integrity, a failure to live up to goals, and even guilt for not doing the 'right thing'. In a study of the social consequences of people who were part of research examining the effectiveness of different weight-reduction diets, some men did not want to acknowledge that they were trying to lose weight to 'look good'. Instead, they believed that they were involved in the study to 'advance science'. Regardless of what the real motive was, this example shows that food and eating convey to eaters something about themselves. And eaters want to convey this image (cultural capital) or identity to the world.

Of course, food is not the only carrier of symbolic capital or social status. One's occupation, place and type of living arrangements have similar functions. However, food is a marker that is easily amenable to change and is often the subject of marketing and promotion on the basis of social status. Food ideas therefore circulate readily as communicators of who we are and also as ways of 'making our selves up', so to speak.

Food and social identity

The ways in which food choices operate to encourage us to belong has been brought out in an interesting study looking at how people with certain body weights tend to seek out people of similar sizes. This has arisen after analysis of social networks within a US community called Framingham, which has been the subject of ongoing medical, health and social examination for many years. Going back over the data on body weight and looking at how social networks change – that is, how people choose who they are going to relate to in friendship and other social circles – researchers found that people who were heavy tended to 'hang out' with others who were of a similar shape. More importantly, the researchers showed that as people became overweight they switched networks so as to form relationships with others who were also overweight. This phenomenon, known as 'social contagion', provides a powerful reminder of the ways in which the results of our food choices allow us to identify with particular social groups and the way that this changes as our body weight changes. The theories behind 'social contagion' are extensive and are not discussed fully here, but are related to the ways in which we feel comfortable in the company of people who we think are more like us. And in the case of larger body size, which increasingly carries social stigma, the need to be part of a group that shares the same experiences and indeed the same justifications is important.

Eating properly as identity

In the same way, the importance placed by some people on eating healthily or 'eating properly' is a powerful signifier of who they are. Indeed, achieving the correct diet, which is an increasing requirement in western culture, has a strong tradition that can be traced back to western antiquity. The main connection here is the way in which cultures place emphasis on making the 'right' choices. In many western cultures that trait can be traced back to Greek antiquity, where this often meant eating in moderation. Indeed, one's food and eating practices were part of a broader concern about how individuals lived their lives. Hubris, or excess, was spurned in ancient Greek culture because it was an indication that self-restraint was lacking, and if you could not control yourself, your chances of controlling your family or estate was unlikely. Therefore your role in contributing to the functioning of Greek society – and we are talking about a society largely ruled by men – was questionable. Thus the relationship between moderation and rationality was struck early in Greek culture. Indeed, one's diet was an extremely important conveyor of one's ability to reason, not only to the wider culture, but as we have seen, to the individuals themselves – their own moral subjectivity. Central to this was the careful management of pleasure, in which, of course, food played an important role.

Coming to more recent times in western culture, we can see how within the dominant religious doctrine food played a major role in creating principles about food. For example, in Christianity food and eating were regarded as ways of strengthening adherence to the faith. Many days were marked out for special dietary practices, whether these were eating particular foods, following particular dietary patterns, or even going without food altogether (fasting). These practices had, and in many cases still have, deep spiritual significance which operated not only to show how outwardly we are part of a particular group, but inwardly how we are able to achieve that membership and what that means to us (joyous, pious, holy). In more modern and secular societies the ability of food to achieve this level of spirituality has weakened. However, many argue that the adherence to diet because of the religious significance has been increasingly replaced in the modern world by another religion: health. Pointing to the fact that 'healthism' is seen by many as a path to inner cleanliness and purity, it is argued that rationality has gradually questioned the basis of religious belief, and the science has emerged as a basis for what to believe in. This transition – that of arguing the basis of religion as health – has a strong tradition, especially as it relates to food. Some popular nineteenth-century promoters of what was considered then to be good healthy eating were also devoutly religious. Their rhetoric was based on achieving spiritual and inner purity through dietary wholesomeness. It is surely not an exaggeration to point to ways in which modern dietary regimes are promoted in ways that are similar: dieting is often regarded as purifying, not only in a bodily sense, but also in a more inner sense – a way of achieving virtue.

Earlier it was mentioned that food provided a basis for belonging to different faiths and followings. It becomes the 'glue' that holds communities and even cultures together. It is this last point, that of culture, to which we now turn in our discussion of food and identity. National cultures are often hallmarked by the so-called 'foodways' the culture has adopted and follows. These cultural foodways become powerful communicators of national identity, which often also extend to geographic identities. Thus, different parts of the same country have affinities with particular foods, ways of food preparation and food patterns; and with that come particular identities. Again, as before, this is not merely a question of showing membership of a culture or a cultural group. It is also a way of creating that food association and constructing one's self – the two-way street. Of course, not all cultures have a strong sense of national and regional food culture, and many would argue that the boundaries have been eroded by a range of developments – from migration to globalisation – all of which have weakened the ties that food has with culture and with cultural membership. But, as is argued here, this does not mean that there is no longer a sense of self about food – or food identity. It means that the food *personalities*, so to speak, have changed and are now experienced along different lines. The example earlier about the subjective experience of eating a Big Mac is an example of this. Big Mac eaters are hardly likely to identify as part of a traditional culture, geographic foodways and cultural groupings. But this does not mean that they are unattached to any cultural grouping and that they are not displaying particular food individualism. It means, instead, that individualism and identity are part of different, wider and more contemporary cultural groupings.

Closing remarks about food and identity

Finally we come to a number of sobering statements. The first is that food *makes* us. That is to say, by virtue of its ability to supply the body with necessary constituents for growth and development, food provides us with a physicality; it constitutes our flesh and bones, all of which provide us with a particular identity. The second statement is that food makes us what we *are*, in the sense that we *are* cultural, social and sentient beings, as well as physical shapes. Food sends powerful messages to us and to others about where we fit culturally and socially. So to say that *you are what you eat* is not a trivial cliché; it is a biological, social and cultural fact.

Further reading

Caplan, P., ed., *Food, Health and Identity*. London: Routledge, 1997.
Christakis, N. and Fowler, J., The spread of obesity in a large social network over 32 years. *New England Journal of Medicine* 357, 370–9, 2007.

Fischler, C., Food, self and identity. *Social Science Information*, 27, 275–92, 1988.

Fischler, C., Commensality, society and culture. *Social Science Information* 1 (50), 528–48, 2011.

Guthman, J., *Weighing In: Obesity, Food Justice and the Limits of Capitalism.* Berkeley, CA: University of California Press, 2011.

Pollock, N., Cultural elaborations of obesity: fattening practices in Pacific societies. *Asia Pacific Journal of Clinical Nutrition* 4, 357–60, 1995.

Porter, R. and Rousseau, G., *Gout: The Patrician Malady.* New Haven, CT: Yale University Press, 1998.

3

FOOD AS ... POLITICS

Introduction

When food and politics are discussed the conversation invariably sits within the realms of food and government (often with a capital G). That is to say, the politics of food is usually concerned with the ways in which government regulation controls the food supply, and the consequences for the public and private interests that prevail in the food supply. The politics of food also invoke discussions of laws and legislation that engage with the food supply. These aspects of food and politics are the focus of future chapters, especially food as regulation and food as industry.

In this chapter the use of the word politics is more nuanced; politics here is taken to mean the ways in which relationships of authority and influence are played out. Thus food politics is concerned with an examination of how food is controlled at different levels. We will start with what I have called 'micro-politics'. Here we will look at how authority and control is exerted at the level of the family, the ways in which family dynamics have changed, and what this means for what is eaten. We will also look at how cooking and cooking skills have been important in exerting certain forms of control at a number of levels. Lastly, we will look at community politics and food, especially the ways in which some initiatives are designed to allow communities and consumers to take control over their food supplies.

Micro-politics of food

During the 1990s I undertook a series of interviews with families to explore the roles food played in family routines and practices. I was particularly interested in how families decided what to eat, how food chores and responsibilities were divided (or not) between family members and how this affected dynamics at the dinner table. At that time there was some interesting research from the UK showing how the taste preferences of the male head of household were paramount in influencing the family mealtimes – if dad loved it, it was on the menu, if not, then no show. In my own research I was trying to find these features in the families I interviewed.

It may have been because of the kinds of families my research attracted, or because the location of my research (Australia) was different from the male-dominated research (UK) or because my approach was not informed by feminism (as was the UK research), or other reasons. But whatever it was, I could not find the patriarchy of the menu that I was expecting. Instead I found a different kind of micro-politics at play in family food and family meal patterns. The most important factors influencing food practices – shopping, cooking, managing meals, juggling food preferences, etc. – in the families I studied were the roles and the place of children. It seemed that children now sat at the top of the table. This finding was confirmed through a pub-lication by other Australian researchers entitled 'Heading the table: parenting and the junior consumer', which describes how children now have a privileged voice on household food matters. To what can we attribute this elevation in children's influence on household food matters? And what are the likely consequences? The next section addresses these issues.

Food, families and children

Like any social grouping, families construct a micro-politics that provides a decision-making process, a sense of governing and way of regulating family life. Central to this is the notion of power and persuasion: Who gets what? How much? Why? This gives rise to establishment of roles and duties. In the families I spoke to in the research mentioned above, discussions focused on how the parents remembered family food dynamics when they were children. Almost without exception, these adults recalled their own childhood times where they were given no choice of what to eat, where food was put in front of them with the expectation that it would be eaten, and, if not, nothing was offered as a substitute. Parents also remembered that meals were often routine, that families had limited budgets and that food was not often wasted. So ideas of thrift, economy and parsimony were common. By their own admission, these conditions did not prevail today. Even the low-income families in my study talked about the relative level of affluence they enjoyed today.

It is an economic fact that as standards of living and incomes increase, so do the range of new markets and opportunities to spend on different goods and services. The food market is no exception. As people in countries like Australia have enjoyed rising affluence, the range and type of foods has burgeoned, and different market segments have developed. One aspect of market segmentation has been the inexorable rise in foods targeting children, with whole sections of the food market now devoted to foods that have child appeal. This has been accompanied by food advertising to children. Marketing to children not only takes place through broadcast media, such as television, but also through non-broadcast media such as the internet. The singling out of children as a market is predicated not only on the fact that children now often have their own disposable income, but also on the interplay between children and parents whereby 'pester power' – the nagging of parents by children for particular goods and services – operates to satisfy children's desires. Parents in my study understood this and said that they tried to control it. But, 'good' parents are also those who support children's wants as well as their needs, so there were plenty of examples where children's whims were pandered to.

However, to point to the arrival of the market segmentation of children as a viable, consuming sub-population with its own wants and needs is to beg the question of how and why children with this set of characteristics arrived in the first place. That is to say, we need to understand the social and political processes through which the role of children in families has changed in order to privilege them as separate, independent and liberated.

In the Australian setting, one of the ways to understand this is through the work of Fallding, whose surveys of family life in the early post-Second World War years revealed interesting changes and developments. Essentially, Fallding's surveys showed that parents were happy to break away from the traditional view of children as 'seen and not heard'. Fallding found quite the opposite: children were now encouraged to speak and parents were encouraged to listen. Indeed, the traditional authoritarian role of parents was being replaced by other roles: the authoritative counsellor (where knowledge was offered not foisted on children); instructive motivator (where horizons were set by parents for children to reach with that knowledge); potential optimiser (where the potential that every child possessed was to be maximised with the right knowledge).

Post-war booming economies in many countries allowed more families to achieve an unprecedented level of affluence. These conditions slowly increased in the 1950s, and noticeably took off in the 1960s and beyond. During that time the role of children changed. Whereas before the Second World War children were often a productive part of the family – often taking on roles and tasks to support family life – in the post-war period children became consumers. The emerging micro-politics in families changed and with that the marketing of a variety of goods and services burgeoned to allow parents to meet the wants and needs of children. And the wants of children took centre stage, as parents of families with fewer children could afford more.

The eventual mix of power in the family is no longer along traditional patriarchal lines, but is much more complex. Children are given much more say about what food is to be eaten in the home and much more choice about food matters. Quite how children arrive at decision-making about the family menu is not clear, but it is more likely to be driven by what is advertised and promoted by food manufacturers than by what is taught as part of the health education programme in schools. The picture is further complicated by new discourses from health professionals about the processes of feeding children, which strongly discourages firmness and insistence by parents at the dinner table. Instead, parents are encouraged to offer food to children with the expectation that if children want to eat it, they will; in other words, parent provides and child decides. However, not only are children's roles and responsibilities in families changing, but also the roles of adults. Women in particular have come under the microscope as domestic responsibilities alter.

Cooking as politics

With predictable regularity there are surveys showing that families are not eating home-cooked food, or are not eating together, or are not eating home-cooked food *and* are not eating together. Reactions to the purported decline in cooking skills are often alarmist, bordering on moral panic. The extent to which a decline in cooking skills is true or based on evidence is actually a moot point, but the very possibility is enough to enliven the imagination and produce dire predictions. Public and professional reactions to the idea that cooking and food preparation skills in families are at risk raises two important questions. First, what is meant by cooking skills; and second, by what standards and measures are they assessed to be adequate? The first question is one that has recently occupied the attention of scholars and policy makers: does cooking mean cooking a meal from scratch, i.e. from the basic ingredients, or pre-prepared foods?

The second question raises the idea of what is a cooked meal and what are the standards by which it is judged to be a proper meal? Research in the UK and Australia beginning in the 1980s found that the 'proper meal' was something familiar to many. Thus cooking a proper meal – often a meal comprising meat, potatoes and vegetables which is often produced as Sunday dinner or similar for a family gathering – is regarded to be the standard against which skills are judged. Proper meals and family meals are often melded and mean similar things. The seriousness of a possible demise of cooking skills has made governments in many countries introduce policies to improve the situation. Community cooking skills programmes have been introduced in community settings for children and adults. Children in Australia now have access to school-based programmes that include growing food gardens and in-school cooking classes where the produce from the garden is turned into meals which the children eat. Elsewhere in schools, traditional home economics classes, which were removed from the curriculum because of a belief in their redundancy, have been replaced by life-skills classes that are heavy with food preparation and cooking practice. The socio-political response to the idea that the modern family is losing skills in food preparation and cooking may be seen as a reaction to and a way of addressing increasing rates of overweight and obesity in industrialised countries, such as the UK and Australia. However, there is possibly a deeper concern at play here, and the evidence for this lies in the fact that widespread government concern about the ability of families to feed themselves 'properly' can be seen in earlier times. For example, the findings in the nineteenth century that led to the growth of nutritional sciences also introduced what was considered to be correct and proper feeding of families. The discovery of food calibration methods that provided measurement of food as calories, or food as protein, also introduced ideas to maximise levels of these ingredients through proper food choices and cooking processes. In the US the work of Wilbur Atwater is probably the best example of this. Atwater's scientific contribution to nutrition is regarded to be out-standing, especially his careful experiments showing that the energy in food when consumed by the human body obeyed the laws of thermodynamics. Atwater's work was driven very much by the political and scientific considerations of the late nineteenth century, with the development of industrial processes in virtually every industry seeking to maximise efficiency (the greatest output) and minimise costs (optimising inputs). Atwater's ground-breaking research had support from a number of social, industrial and political quarters. The US government funded his research and laboratories were established in a number of universities. Industrial interest and support from captains of business arose from Atwater's development of a calculation of the food needs of humans, which were converted to so-called 'pecuniary needs'; that is the cost of feeding humans according to their basic physiology requirements – literally, the cost of living. Given that food costs comprised the biggest item in the family budget, basing the cost of living and thus a living wage on pecuniary needs is a powerful argument to make. Thus US industrialists of the day were quick to use Atwater's findings to counter trade union claims of what a reasonable cost of living might be. The scientific logic of eating according to physiological 'needs' rather than 'wants' was very persuasive. Atwater and colleagues went to great lengths to publicise how families could meet their physiological needs (calories, grams of protein, etc.) in the most economical manner, and magazines and almanacs carried tables and ready reckoners of the costs of different foods that provided maximum amounts of basic nutrients. Interestingly, Atwater was scathing about the consumption of fruits and vegetables, which he believed to be an indulgence and wasteful because they contained little energy or protein compared to foods with less water content, such as grains. Writing before the discovery of vitamins and other plant-based nutrients, his work is a sobering reminder of the implications of the limits of knowledge and understanding. Socially, Atwater's work gained popularity among church and other faith-based groups who were engaged in works of charity with the less fortunate social classes. Armed with the scientific logic of nutrition and ways in which 'proper' eating – that is, maximising energy and protein intake while minimising expenditure – could be undertaken, charity workers could engage even more forcefully with the groups they were serving. The work of Atwater also instigated social movements that sought to improve community cooking skills that could now be based on science, rather than tradition or custom. The development of domestic science, later known as home science or home economics, was a natural consequence of the application of Atwater's work on food and nutrition. And the later introduction of home science into schools in many countries, such as the US, UK and Australia mostly, of course, to girls – was justified by the need to teach 'proper', that is science-based, cooking skills and other domestic duties.

Food politics and national security

Another period where the vulnerability of population health and welfare could be at risk because of poor cooking and food preparation skills can be found during the Second World War, especially in countries like the UK. The national emergency brought about by chronic food shortages due to the vulnerability of food imports, especially from the US, triggered a government response that was far reaching and indeed, for many, far sighted. The UK ration system, which underpinned the maintenance of food security, was founded on scientific principles. Drawing on Atwater's work and that of discoveries of nutritional scientists who worked in the earlier part of the twentieth century, food was rationed according to the physiological needs of babies, children, pregnant and lactating women, and adult men and women. The government sought to maximise the use of rationed and other food through programmes and propaganda encouraging cooking skills based on economy and waste minimisation. Recipe development using ingredients that were easy to access, rather than tradition or convention, became part of the 'war effort' and austerity became a virtue.

Coming to the present, we can see that the importance given to shoring up what are to be cooking skills shortages depends very much on a context of vulnerability. In Atwater's time this vulnerability arose because of a perception that maximum use of food nutrients had been overlooked because of an ignorance of scientific facts. In the case of the Second World War, the vulnerability resulted from imminent national food insecurity. Today it may be argued that the vulnerability stems from rising levels of diet-related chronic diseases. This, however, is only part of the picture. Arguing from the obvious point that panics over cooking skills result in women being the targets of programmes and campaigns to address the decline, we might say that the concern is more about the changing role of women in domestic and social life. Certainly there is plenty of popular and professional literature that purports to show how women moving out of the home into paid employment has created a so—called vulnerability in domestic food security. The reliance by households on pre-prepared foods, which are regarded to be less nutritious, more energy-dense, etc. is regarded to be a consequence of this development. Thus food is itrinsic to the dynamics of domestic political life.

Food politics in the community

If food can be a catalyst for politics within the home, recent developments have shown that food can also be a rallying call for the community. The move towards communities coming together around food issues has become a feature of many advanced capitalist economies. Whether this is out of a suspicion of increasing modernity and the increasing intrusion of industry or business in everyday life, or whether out of a legacy of the virtuous frugality brought about by the austere measures introduced during the Second World War, or whether as part of a resistance to change arising from the counter culture of the 1960s, it is hard to say. Certainly the aims of food movements have different roots and refer to different constituencies; however, they may be usefully summarised as supporting alternative food systems that maximise human involvement and engagement and minimise industrial impact and degradation of the environment. Alternative to what, you might ask? The main concerns that foster alternative food movements focus on *Big Food*, which, similar to juggernauts like *Big Oil* or *Big Banks*, is a motif for increased concentration and power in the food supply. These new alternative food sectors come in many shapes and sizes.

Farmers' markets

Over the past 20 years more than 3,500 new farmers' markets have emerged in the US. In the UK that number is about 450. Farmers' market provide an opportunity for consumers to buy directly from producers – farmers or agricultural producers. This essentially eliminates the retail sector, especially supermarkets. Politically this is a loud statement since supermarkets are often the most powerful players in the food chain, so being able to circumvent them is very much a political act. By virtue of missing the 'middle man', farmers' markets also reduce the distance travelled by food from production to consumption, often referred to as 'food miles'. Reducing food miles between producers and consumers reduces the use of fossil fuels, which highlights concerns about the environmental effects of greenhouse gas emissions.

Food, place and politics

Living on low food miles has had another effect. It has given rise to the notion of the 'locavore'. This is someone who eats food grown and produced within a particular and defined food geography, such as within a 100-mile radius. Eating locally and seasonally has also given impetus to another food trend known as community supported agriculture (CSA), where consumers develop close relationships with primary producers from whom they buy food directly. CSAs also support the inclusion of consumers in the agricultural tasks required to grow food. So CSA farms invite their consumer members to attend at weekends and take part in nurturing the very act of food production. Again, these initiatives send powerful political messages. Not only are environmental and nutritional issues addressed (low food miles, emphasis on fresh, unprocessed foods, etc.), but also ideological positions are vindicated. Some citizens have taken a further step; they have established themselves as food producers.

Over the past five years there has been a steady increase in the emphasis on home or backyard food gardening. In many countries this is not exactly new. In the UK, for example, allotments – small patches of council land released for growing food or flowers – have been made available. The backyard food production movement worldwide was given great prominence when, on moving into the White House, one of Michelle Obama's first actions was to dig up a large area for an urban food garden. Many have seen this act to be less about food provisioning and more about what is known as food democracy. Food democracy has emerged as a highly political idea. It represents the way in which citizens can take back at least some control of their food supply. Growing your own food means not eating someone else's. It also allows an appreciation of food provenance. In Australia, the importance of food gardening, especially as a way of teaching children to appreciate the provenance of food, can be seen in a national campaign initiative by celebrity chef Stephanie Alexander. After the success of a demonstration project kitchen garden in an inner-city Melbourne primary school, the Stephanie Alexander Kitchen Garden programme went nationwide, supported by over 12.5 million dollars of public funding.

Closing remarks about food as politics

Food provides us with a sharp vision about the ways in which political arrangements exist at the micro and macro levels. Looking at how food politics operates in families effectively shows us how power relationships exist. In contrast to the usual understandings of power, in which domination is assumed, what is clear with food are the complex ways in which rules are produced and reproduced to allow certain functions to be performed. At the community level power also exists. However, the power of the *idea* of community food systems – which brings home to conventional food systems many of the problems that the food supply now faces – is immense.

Further reading

Aronson, N., Nutrition as a social problem: A case study of entrepreneurial strategy in science. *Social Problems* 29: 474–87, 1982.

Attar, D., *Wasting Girls' Time: The History and Politics of Home Economics*. London: Virago, 1990.

Charles, N. and Kerr, M., *Women, Food and Families*. Manchester: Manchester University Press, 1988.

Cottingham, L., *The Taste of War: World War Two and the Battle for Food*. London: Allen Lane, 2011.

DeVault, M., *Feeding the Family: The Social Organisation of Caring as Gendered Work*. Chicago, IL: University of Chicago Press. 1991.

Short, F. *Kitchen Secrets: The Meaning of Cooking in Everyday Life*. New York: Berg Publishers, 2006.

4

FOOD AS ... INDUSTRY

Introduction

This chapter will examine the ways in which the lens of food provides us with an insight into the processes of commodification of food. That is to say, how food becomes a product that is sold, bought and consumed. The dynamic nature of the food market is such that we will see how there have been major developments in a relatively short space of time. The reasons behind these developments will be explored. The food industry has been the subject of much work by a wide range of people, and indeed this whole book could be taken up with an examination of this fascinating subject. The purpose of this chapter is, however, not to explore the whole of the industrialised food chain and the players in it. It is more to see how food provides us with a particular insight into the business – indeed big business – of food.

Food producers and consumers

Some time ago I spent two years working and living in Papua New Guinea. One of my early observations was that most people in rural areas were entirely self-sufficient. In their food gardens they grew the foods they ate and had no need to buy any more. Sometimes they hunted or fished for food and, occasionally, went on food-gathering expeditions to collect food from trees and bushes, or dig it up from the earth.

For Papua New Guineans in the towns, however, the story was entirely different. They would buy weekly supplies of food from fresh-food markets and shop in supermarkets for meat, fish and other commodities. In other words, for town people there was a gap between food producers and consumers. The Papua New Guinea story is an example of a trend that has been happening in most cultures for many years; indeed, self-sufficiency is very rare and most people rely on others to produce food for them.

The growing gap between food producers and food consumers has been a cause of concern. Relinquishing control of one's food supply appears to create a level of anxiety that indicates how important food connections are. For example, the lack of knowledge of the provenance of food, its origins, methods of production, and forms of labour are regarded as factors contributing to a number of problems – from being overweight to contributing to greenhouse gas emissions. Stories that are expected to 'shock' abound – for example, children believing that milk comes from cartons, not cows; shoppers expecting foods out of season; consumers not knowing what key ingredients comprise even the most basic foods. All this suggests that there is something fundamental about the need to know where our food comes from, and how it got onto our plate. Much of the discussion – some would say blame – concerns the rise of an industry that developed to mass produce and mass market our food. It is an industry on which most of us rely on a daily basis.

Of course, in most cultures there have always been some industries in food supply, in other words, people and businesses charged with the responsibility of making particular food products, whether this be bread, cheese, meat products, etc. These industries developed as specialisations in response to the need to supply communities with foods that people could not, or did not want to, supply for themselves. In many countries and cultures these industries still exist and, for a large part, are revered for the traditions they uphold. For example, French culture places a lot of value on regional foods that are manufactured by local, often small, industries. It is the size of these industries and their connection with the local culture and local geography that makes them attractive. In Australia, and some other western countries, there has been a revival of such industries, albeit in a way that is often described as artisanal, registering that the producers are more like craftspeople than mass marketers. So the concerns about separation of food producers and consumers are not about food industries *per se*, but more the scale and size. The term *Big Food* has been used to describe a particular type of enterprise, which is often seen to be megalithic in terms of representing an interlocking system, and monolithic in terms of magnitude.

Big Food

The development of *Big Food* is an issue of contention. Some argue that the rise in *Big Food* developed in response to increasing urbanisation. Indeed, the town dwellers in Papua New Guinea are a clear example of the trends towards urban living seen in many places around the world. This trend started much earlier in many western cultures. In the UK, for example, it is argued that since the late eighteenth century there has been the movement of people from rural areas to towns. This gave rise to the need for urban populations to have access to food that they could no longer grow or supply for themselves.

This argument assumes that, in fact, in the rural setting people were able to subsist on supplies that they themselves created, whereas, as noted earlier, it is highly likely that local food systems were the mainstay of the rural food supply. Also, urbanisation by itself does not necessarily herald an industrial food supply, as suggested by *Big Food*. In a number of European cultures, urbanised populations were serviced by small companies that were not highly industrial.

Some authors have argued that there was a fundamental shift in food-supply thinking during and after the Second World War. For example, Lang and Heasman suggest that the threats to food security at this time gave rise to a different form of food production and distribution. They use the term 'food productionism' to describe how food-systems thinking in the UK, for example, prioritised growing and producing more food. Food productionism is not merely about more food, however. It is about a system that provides more food, one that is intensified, industrialised and increasingly concentrated. The key terms here are yield, throughput and profitability.

Thus at the primary production end the system requires 'inputs', such as fertilisers, pesticides and herbicides, to assist growth and maturation of raw materials, like crops. It requires veterinary drugs to protect animals from communicable diseases. In some jurisdictions it requires animal growth promoters to hasten the time taken for animal maturation and market readiness. Further down the chain, the primary sector such as farms, abattoirs and mills needed to be rationalised and integrated, and larger companies became responsible for fewer products. The necessary preservation of food that is being mass-produced requires secondary processing, such as canning, drying, freezing, etc. To retain some of the features of the unprocessed product – or even to exaggerate these – processing often included the addition of colourings, flavourings and preservatives.

As Lang and Heasman point out, the results of this intensification and industrialisation has been impressive and mostly positive. With more mouths to feed in post-war economies, food productionism was able to deliver more food and, indeed, cheaper food. However, food productionism tends to lead to overproduction and even stockpiling; it thus needs a counterpart if its economic viability is to be realised. This counterpart developed in what might be called food consumptionism – that is, a range of industries whose job is to encourage food consumption way beyond the level of need and subsistence.

Food consumptionism is not a lone entity, but may be seen as part of a growing culture of consumption in post-Second World War economies, where economic growth and prosperity were being enjoyed on many fronts. 'Mass marketing', whether for cars, fridges, clothes or food, was the name given to this phenomenon. And the place for mass marketing is the high streets and shopping centres – what George Ritzler calls the 'Cathedrals of consumption'. Consumption has become so embedded in everyday social existence that some suggest that it has replaced religion as 'the dominant mode of contemporary public life'.

Jane Dixon and colleagues have used the term 'consumptogenic environments' to describe the situations and settings that compel us to consume. These environments have a number of characteristics. First, they are environments where goods and services are relentlessly promoted and advertised. Indeed, the industries that accompany consumptogenic environments, such as marketing and advertising, spend a fortune working on ways to encourage consumers to forget their needs and focus on their wants.

Second, they are environments devoid of any sense of restriction, parsimony or self-restraint. Indeed, anything that smacked of 'going without' is seen as almost pathological; 'Want it – have it' is the credo. Thus the description of these environments as cathedrals of consumption is entirely apt. Finally, these environments promote the attainment of pleasure as the ultimate goal of self-fulfilment. In a sense there is a deliberate blurring of pleasure-seeking with happiness-seeking. The former is marketed as the result of acquiring various trappings that are believed to satisfy some form of gratification, which then is supposed to lead to happiness and self-fulfilment. However, this is a very tenuous relationship, especially when the marketing of goods and services is often based on fostering and inculcating a deep unhappiness in individuals about themselves. That is to say, much promotion is focused on human flaws and vulnerabilities that are expected to be removed through the acquisition of whatever is being pushed. Mostly the satisfaction of one's wants does not lead to the fulfilment of one's happiness, as many studies have shown. Nevertheless, so successful is the food productionism–food consumptionism relationship that the amount of food bought and not used is immense. Indeed, the quantity of wasted food has now reached vast amounts. The telling aspect of this is that – according to our current knowledge – the largest component of food waste is at the level of the household. In other words, a significant amount of the food that is brought into most households ends up in the bin. So the measure of success of *Big Food* is its ability to produce food and promote its consumption. A look at the exact nature of *Big Food* will help us understand why.

The dimensions of *Big Food*

There is some contention as to what exactly *Big Food* is. Some define it only as the ubiquitous 'fast-food' market, a definition that focuses only on the big multinational takeaway chains such as MacDonald's, KFC, Burger King, etc. Certainly the global proliferation of these chains can be regarded as an example of the mass marketing of food. As they set up shop in a range of cultures, fast-food businesses do not always merely import what they sell 'back home'. The process known as 'glocalisation' describes the ways in which fast-food outlets embrace local ingredients and even local cultures. For example, in Sydney, the suburb of Lakemba is renowned for the size of the Islamic population. The local fast-food restaurants and ones in neighbouring suburbs adapted their menus accordingly by promoting halal versions of their popular offerings.

However, other examples of *Big Food* refer to the growth of not only fast food, but also the spread of supermarkets and hypermarkets, many of which stock up to 15,000–20,000 different food items.

Indeed, it is the central role played by this retail sector that, in the eyes of many, is the heart and soul of *Big Food*. This is because supermarket retailers, such as large chains, are the interface of production and consumption. Thus supermarket retailers are in a very powerful position. They have purchasing desks where decisions are made about what lines are going to be carried and what products are going to appear on shelves. Manufacturers have to compete with each other to get their products into supermarkets and onto the most prominent places where they have the greatest visibility. It is not uncommon to see a line of products, say bread, biscuits or tinned tomatoes, with perhaps ten different manufacturers represented. It is sobering to also remember that probably at least another ten manufacturers' products do not appear for sale because the supermarket chain's purchasing desk decided not to accommodate these lines.

The big players in *Big Food*

The power of large supermarket chains in choice editing and negotiating prices is probably seen most visibly in the fresh-food sector. Here, food producers contract with supermarkets to take their crop, harvest or yield, depending on what is being produced. This contract virtually locks in producers to the supermarket, allowing the chain to negotiate very low prices to the producer. These low prices are often settled even before the crop has been harvested, and there have been many concerns about the fact that the settled price is too low for producers to make a living. The phenomenon is especially acute when supermarket chains begin so-called 'price wars'. For example, in Australia fresh milk price wars have been raging. One supermarket chain has reduced the price of its fresh milk to a level which is below the cost of production. That is to say, the cost of producing milk is greater than the price for which farmers are selling it to super-markets. This, of course, means that the farmers are losing money. However, while this might lead to fewer dairy farms in the business, because they are going broke, it does not mean there are fewer cows. This is because larger dairy companies can take over as farmers sell out. Thus we see larger dairy mono-polies, by virtue of the economies of scale, absorbing some of the cost/price issues that individual farmers cannot. This form of so-called 'vertical integration', whereby large supermarket chains deal with large food-producing monopolies, is another feature of *Big Food*.

But does any of this really matter to the consumer, who in the end benefits from lower prices? What concern is it of consumers whether, for example, their milk comes from Fred's dairy or from Dairy Industries Pty Ltd? Surely, as long as the milk is fresh, pure, of consistent quality, isn't that all that matters to people actually buying the product? In the short term, the answer is perhaps 'yes'. Consumers are not always fussy about the 'upstream factors' that play out in the food chain, only the price and quality of what is on the shelves. Mostly, shoppers shoulder a significant number of household and, increasingly, employment responsibilities, and do not want to be troubled by the economics behind the food supply. However, the consumer may lose out in the end. This is because once the larger companies have a monopoly, then competition in the marketplace suffers. For example, there is a belief that the Australian milk pricing war mentioned earlier will eventually lead to the disappearance of the fresh milk market, leaving long–life(UHT) cartoned milk as the only option available for consumers. This is already the case in many countries, where fresh milk has become something of a boutique commodity.

So far the scale and size of *Big Food* has an overall effect on the market. But what are the health consequences of *Big Food*?

Big Food and health

Can we be clearer about what is the major concern with Big Food? After all, if *Big Food* is bringing us cheaper foods and cheaper ingredients from which we can make meals and dishes, can this not be a good thing?

There is much debate as to what actually is the concern about *Big Food*. Some people, for example Carlos Monteiro, have separated foods into three groups. First is whole or unprocessed foods, a category that perhaps speaks for itself. These are foods that are largely as nature intended: fresh fruits and vegetables, wholegrain products with minimal processing. Next are processed culinary ingredients, such as oil, flour, sugar. These are foods that have for hundreds of years been part of a food processing industry, albeit small and local in some places.

Then there is what are called ultra-processed foods. These are foods that have proliferated in the late twentieth and early twenty-first centuries and comprise the majority of products that can be considered as snack foods, ready-to-eat foods and pre-prepared foods. The sale of ultra-processed foods has exploded in many countries, and not just the wealthy ones. Many believe that these foods, by virtue of their low cost, high availability and high energy density (that is, calories per gram), are responsible for the so-called 'obesity epidemic' that is being seen across the world. The growth of ultra-processed foods is not an accident. There are a number of push and pull factors that have created a market and a place for them in many homes, which some say would be hard put to do without them. The pull factors might be described as the changing work–life balance many households have experienced. This has been brought about by a number of factors, including the movement of women into paid employment, where they are often holding down a number of part-time jobs. Some see the availability of part-time work as resulting from another development, that is the casualisation of the labour market.

The result is that whereas women were most likely to take responsibility for household food procurement and preparation, that role is now more precariously filled. It is true that, as surveys show, women still shoulder the responsibility of shopping and cooking, but with pressures in the casualised labour market, there is less time to prepare food, and the use of ultra-processed foods has been the result. Another pull factor is the acceptance by family members of foods that have been formulated to be highly palatable, of consistent quality, high availability, affordability and convenience. This last point refers to the fact that ultra-processed foods rarely, if ever, require any cooking skills to produce meals. Thus the time and trouble of food preparation is spared.

Whether the increased use of ultra-processed foods has in fact led to a decrease in cooking is a question that is very contentious, and the proposition that cooking in households has been declining is being hotly debated, as we saw in the previous chapter. This brings us to the push factors that have made ultra-processed foods popular. Probably chief among these is aggressive and highly visible marketing and promotion through multiple media sources. Highly processed, easy to prepare, convenient and economical food now comprises the majority of food products advertised on television, radio and other mass media sources. Their place on the family menu and their warm reception by family members is a familiar and successful promotion and selling point. Watch any television advertisement for an example of families enthusiastically lapping up the latest to be marketed easy-to-prepare product.

Another push factor is the high palatability of ultra-processed foods. Pre-market testing ensures that they are flavoursome and appetising, or at least not unappetising. Of course, taste and flavour are always a matter of individual preference, but the sheer popularity of ultra-processed foods attests to the fact that they 'hit the spot' for many. This often means they are high in ingredients that convey flavour, such as salt, sugar (or syrups) or fat, or indeed, in the case of some ultra-processed foods, all three. They also attempt to look appealing by virtue of ingredients to improve visual impact, such as colourings. So the immediate push factors are things like heavy marketing of attractive foods, which are promoted to slot straight into a family setting with minimum fuss and maximum appeal. There is another push factor that is important here: price. Ultra-processed foods are usually competitively priced and are promoted as such.

There are many consequences of these push and pull factors that need to be considered. Some have already been mentioned, such as a possible drop in occasions when households cook, and the possible disappearance of cooking skills. This development is causing a number of worries, especially because of the belief that children will not be exposed in the home to the opportunities to cook, or at least to see someone else cooking.

Another concern is that, because many ultra-processed foods are directly marketed to children, especially young children, there is a likelihood that children will be exploited due to their gullibility and credulity in images and scenarios promoted in food advertising. Another concern is that children will develop a preference for these foods to the detriment of their health. The World Health Organization has made the link between the heavy marketing of ultra-processed foods – so-called junk foods – and rising rates of childhood obesity.

A third concern is that because of the low cost and high convenience of ultra-processed foods, fresh minimally processed foods will become a rare ingredient in family foods and dishes. Indeed, there have been a number of studies showing that fresher, healthier foods – especially fruits and vegetables, but also lower-fat food varieties – are in fact comparatively expensive. What is more, fresher foods are often fragile, with a limited shelf life. This is on top of the fact that fresher ingredients require preparation in the conversion into edible dishes that will be acceptable to families. Whereas ultra-processed foods, by virtue of pre-market testing, competitive pricing and heavy advertising, will have greater appeal.

Food as industry ... what does it tell us?

So what does a food lens provide us with when looking at advancing industrialisation? Three important issues are made clear. First, the opening remarks about the move in Papua New Guinea to urbanisation, and the need for consumers to rely on others to produce food also indicates changes in not just people's lifestyles, but in national economies. These changes are happening around the world, and few places have remained unaffected. Food gives us a chance to see how these changes are played out in everyday practices, and what the likely consequences are. It is hard to see a return to a time when households have a 'food manager', usually the mother, whose role is to convert raw ingredients into family meals on a regular basis. So the examination of 'food as industry' also shows us how roles within the family have changed and how these changes cement our relationship with, indeed our reliance on, industry. Indeed, some would see industrial sources of food as liberating women and releasing them from their domestic role in the home.

The second issue that food as industry throws light on are the ways in which market forces and dynamics change, often very rapidly. The manufacturing part of any commodity sector has traditionally been seen as the 'engine' of the industry, which assumes that the market is mostly under the influence of what is being produced and manufactured. However, recent changes in the food industry demonstrate that food producers and manufacturers are in many ways less powerful than the retail sector. Large supermarket chains have grown to become major players in the field, wielding enormous power. In her book on the changing role of chicken in the food economy, Jane Dixon shows how moving from frozen to chilled chicken allowed food retailers to take the lead on what foods were offered for sale to consumers. Retailers were then able to dominate the chicken producers about what was required and what customers wanted. The move from manufacturer- to retailer-driven markets is a trend that may be followed in other commodities.

It is true that growing concerns about the impact of *Big Food*, which go back to the 1960s, have given rise to a number of what are called 'alternative to commercial' food systems. These systems have enjoyed growing popularity. They embrace initiatives such as farmers' markets, where consumers can shop and buy directly from producers. Also in this category are box schemes, which provide consumers with weekly boxes of fresh food comprising produce that has been directly sourced from producers. These schemes often promote organic foods, or foods that are locally grown. Another alternative to the commercial food system are community food gardens and food swaps. The latter consists of regular events where householders can take food grown in their own garden, often an overabundance, and swap it for that grown by others. Community food gardens now proliferated so that local governments or councils are actively supporting them. Finally, in this group we can place school food and garden schemes. These have developed in response to the concern that children might not have an opportunity to witness the gardening of fresh fruit and vegetables, or the preparation of food and dishes from raw or at least minimally processed ingredients. Commonly, schools will set aside a patch for a food garden and children have the responsibility for planting and maintaining the food grown. Moreover, children get to harvest the food when ready and take it into the classroom/kitchen, where they can assist in the preparation of dishes, and finally eat meals prepared from such food harvested.

Finally, the food as industry lens shows that the production side of the commodity is matched by the consumption drivers of the economy. The marketing of food – advertising and other promotional activities – has burgeoned. Consumption is driven by very savvy and slick campaigns. More recently the influence of broadcast media, especially cooking shows and 'celebrity chef' programmes, may have played a role. The academic literature in this area is not well developed, but other indicators are that cooking programmes, such as reality television shows like Masterchef and Junior Masterchef, can tie in with supermarkets and achieve top viewer ratings.

Closing remarks on food as industry

The complexity of capitalist industrial processes are well captured when viewed through food. The food industry and its regulation show us how institutions, both private and public, shape and are shaped by our social lives and everyday practices. Some might say that we have the food industry we deserve. It is one that has responded well to the changes in lifestyles, work patterns and family relationships. Of concern is the extent to which individuals and families have control over their food habits. With the development and sophistication of marketing and advertising, there is the problem of overconsumption and its consequences. This is an issue we look at in the next chapter.

Further reading

Carolan, M., *The Real Cost of Cheap Food*. Abingdon: Earthscan, 2011.
Dixon, J., *Changing Chicken: Chooks, Cooks and Culinary Culture*. Sydney: University of New South Wales Press, 2002.

Lang, T. and Heasman, M., *Food Wars: The Battle for Mouths, Minds and Markets*. London: Earthscan, 2004.

Monteiro, C., The big issue is ultra-processing. *Journal of the World Public Health Nutrition Association* 1 (6), 237–69, 2010.

Pollan, M., *The Omnivore's Dilemma: A Natural History of Four Meals*. London: Penguin, 2007.

Roberts, P., *The End of Food*. Boston, MA: Mariner Books, 2008.

5

FOOD AS ... REGULATION

Introduction

The purpose of this book is to demonstrate that using food as a lens, we can examine important issues that have impacted our human development. This chapter looks at the notion of government and regulation. These directives, both together and separately, have become important aspects of human societies. And food has played a crucial role in this.

We begin by looking at some aspects of food that we often take for granted – the role of legislation to provide for us a food supply which is clean (largely), safe (mostly) and reliable (in most cases). We then look at other factors that have regulated our appetites for food, particularly social, cultural and religious practices. Finally we look at how, more recently, the idea of self-regulation – a very old concept in many cultures – has developed in response to rising levels of affluence and accompanying practices of excess.

Regulation and the need for safe food

It is easy to think of examples where our food supply has simply failed to deliver in terms of providing food that is safe, clean and reliable. It is important to be aware, however, of how our food supply has improved, notwithstanding our nostalgia for what we think were earlier, simpler times when food was less processed and less complicated. However, it is sobering to remember that, even less than 150 years ago, the food supply in many countries was not safe, was not clean and certainly was not reliable. This is true today, of course, for many countries in less developed parts of the world.

It was the introduction of major and significant pieces of legislation during the middle of the nineteenth century in countries such as the UK and Australia that created a whole new landscape for regulation of food and food safety. Food regulation was one of the first pieces of public health law to be introduced in many countries. Indeed, the very first law passed in Port Jackson, the earliest Australian colonial settlement (later named Sydney), was one to regulate clean drinking water from a stream that was the colony's main water supply.

It was rampant food defilement – in the growing industrial nineteenth-century towns of Europe, but also common in rural areas too – that brought about a need for food laws to prohibit adulteration, dilution and other forms of contamination. The Pure Food Act was passed by the UK parliament in 1860, and with this came the need to police the food supply for cases of breaching or violating. The Act was changed and updated regularly so it could keep pace with changing food processing practices by food companies, large and small. With the increasing role played by food manufacturers, where food-processing techniques were being introduced, so came the need to apply regulation and legislation to ensure that the processed food was not harmful to health and not likely to deceive consumers.

The exercise of some kind of control over the food supply has a longer history. One of the earliest examples of a law on food purity can be found as far back as 1266 in the form of the *Assize on Bread*, a law introduced by King John of England to govern the weight and price of bread. This was updated regularly until as late as 1822, after which a Bread Act was introduced to govern bread prices and the weight of loaves.

As the food supply became more industrialised, and the distance between producers and consumers became bigger, the need to introduce more laws and regulations increased. In Australia, food regulation involves a number of federal, state and local government organisations who each play a role in keeping the food supply clean, safe and reliable.

Occasionally there are breaches in the safety of food, which have been highly publicised. The development in the UK of bovine spongiform encephalopathy (BSE or 'mad cow disease') is one of the most famous, and changed the course of food legislation and regulation across many countries. Even in places such as Australia, which was never found to have any cases of BSE, legislation was introduced to protect the food supply from possible contamination. Australia has had its own food contamination problems: the case of Garibaldi metwurst (cooked sausage) in South Australia is one of the most well known. Here, problems with the processing of metwurst, a processed meat that is usually fermented and not cooked, allowed toxic contaminants to remain in the product, causing the deaths of some children who consumed the product. More recently, contamination with melamine of milk and milk products imported into Australia from China received public scrutiny.

A major outcome of the regulation and legislation of the food supply – and the public awareness of food safety – has presented a sense of risk and caution for individuals, communities and wider populations. Research has shown that in many countries consumer fears about the quality and safety of food are substantial, and media reporting of yet another scare or scandal serves to heighten concerns. Notwithstanding this, regulation of the food supply is often taken for granted. Not unreasonably, the public expect government and industry checks and balances to be in place to keep food safe and of high quality. Indeed, so ingrained is this expectation that research shows most people place almost blind faith in food regulation and hardly ever consider it a problem unless a scare or scandal breaks out.

Regulation and culture

Of course, it would be wrong to believe that before the introduction of food laws and legislation people ate in a willy-nilly fashion. Throughout history what was eaten was usually governed by what was available, and historically, for a large part of the population, food supplies were precarious. Natural disasters like pestilence, crop failure and diseases in beasts destined for the table created a food supply that was for the most part unreliable. Hunger, even starvation, was common. Of course, for sections of society that were more affluent food supplies were more predictable, but not unregulated; there were often rules that governed what was eaten. Sumptuary laws were common in the European Middle Ages to regulate a range of consumption practices. One of these was food. Rules borrowed from laws of the church provided a number of strictures on what food could be eaten and when. In Christianity there were rules about when meat could be eaten, and when it should be eschewed. In other cultures, such as Islam, rules existed about the avoidance of flesh from the pig, as is also the case in Judaism, where a number of other dietary restrictions are applied, informed by the edicts laid out in the Old Testament, especially the Book of Leviticus. Other religions such as Buddhism and Hinduism have dietary rules. All this is to say that the relationship humans have with food has generally been regulated in one form or another, and that what is eaten is a matter of culture, governed by social mores, customs and traditions, as well as nature, which governs what the body needs by way of nutrients.

The rise in self-regulation

There have been a number of recent social transitions, starting initially in more affluent countries, but now spreading across the globe, concerned with the nature of individual food regulation and self-governance of appetite. As mentioned earlier, much of what people were able to eat was regulated by what and how much food was available. Even as the food supply became industrialised, and food supplies more secure, there were limits on the amount of food available for households to consume, often because of affordability of food. For example, until recently for most households in the UK and Australia household expenditure on food was the highest item in the family budget. In some cases more than 60 per cent of household expenditure was on food. During the post-Second World War period a number of developments happened to change this. First, food became cheaper, as was explained in Chapter 4. This was due to the introduction of what has been termed food productionism, where the overall amount of food grown, processed and available for sale increased massively. However, a second factor simply made food more affordable for many households. This was due to increases in household income with the move from single to dual incomes in many households. Thus, lower food prices and increased household income – and thus greater spending power – led to more food being eaten.

Overall, the rise in affluence created conditions that were conducive to better health and wellbeing. Most households could afford a number of goods and services that made a substantial difference to better-quality lifestyles and personal habits. These ranged from being able to afford to live in homes in healthier districts or suburbs (with more and bigger bedrooms, which reduced overcrowding and spread of infectious diseases), to better sanitation (with more accessible household ablution facilities), to cleaner clothes (better cleaning agents and, in many cases, washing machines), to eating more and better food. Also, a number of effective public health measures were made more available, such as immunisation for babies and children. Throughout the 1950s and 1960s in countries like Australia, rising affluence and better standards of living were simply taken for granted.

Regulating affluence

The effects of affluence on lifestyles, especially increased sedentary behaviour along with increasing food intake, are thought to have caused an increase in a number of conditions that were labelled as 'lifestyle' diseases. Chief among these are cardiovascular diseases such as heart disease and stroke. The links between affluent lifestyles and so-called chronic diseases were strengthened by epidemiology showing that these diseases were virtually absent from populations living more traditional lifestyles, such as New Guinea Highlanders and African Bantu.

From the 1960s to the present, medical science and epidemiology have revealed a number of dietary lifestyle diseases, from bowel problems arising because of low dietary fibre, to forms of cancer due to low intakes of fruit and vegetables, to cardiovascular disease due to high intakes of saturated fats. Many attribute the increase in diet-related diseases to a greater reliance on so-called 'convenience' foods, which are a product of growing affluence. While these foods – which by their very nature have been processed and pre-prepared – have reduced the time needed for preparation and transformation into family meals, they often have high levels of fat, sugar, salt, and are low in dietary fibre. Thus the prosperity and affluence that brought better health comes with a sting in the tail: too much of a good thing.

As a way of addressing lifestyle diseases, governments and medical authorities have introduced measures designed to problematise affluent lifestyles, by encouraging people to be more physically active, and to prepare food from basic ingredients and overall eat less. These dietary measures to make populations healthy are entirely different from those that existed in earlier times, where regulation, legislation and laws sought to make the food environment cleaner and safer. The current measures are about another kind of regulation: self-regulation. In other words, individuals are targeted with information and advice about how to make changes in their dietary choices, and their physical activity. The tone of health advice suggests that people should show restraint in lifestyle habits: eat less, exercise more. Using strategies borrowed from the commercial sector, social marketing campaigns are launched to encourage dietary change and patterns of physical activity. Little acknowledgement is given, however, to the current social context, where 'consumptogenesis' is rife. In the previous chapter we were introduced to the idea of a consumptogenic environment that is fed by push factors such as heavy advertising and marketing, and pull factors such as affluence and sedentary lifestyles. Within this environment any expectation that people can meaningfully self-regulate is entirely misplaced.

Most western cultures have foregone any sense of self-denial or restraint. For example, unlike many cultures that routinely practise some form of dietary restraint associated with a religious calendar, such as Ramadan in Islam, or routine fasting in Hinduism or Buddhism, no such events occur in the cultural calendar of the majority of populations living in the UK, US or Australia. The period of Lent – where some form of pleasure or gratification is foregone for the 40 days from the Tuesday before Ash Wednesday (Mardi Gras) until Easter Sunday – is no longer recognised except for a few European countries. For most of us, Easter is regarded to be just another time to consume more, whether this is hot cross buns or Easter eggs. All this is to say that regulation of individual appetites is extremely difficult, relying as it does on individual self-denial without any form of support from religious or other cultural practices. Restraint has no place in consumptogenic environments, which promise that the more we consume the happier we will be. Even though we know from the work of people like Clive Hamilton and Richard Denniss that this is not so. They use the term *Affluenza* to describe a condition whereby people consuming more, actually leads to less: less enchantment, less happiness and less fulfilment.

We have seen so far that the imperative to exercise some form of regulation over individual appetites has a legacy in many cultures. Michel Foucault, in his volumes on the *History of Sexuality*, addresses the ways in which the regulation of sexual activities has been practised in western cultures. Today, sex is highly regulated: who one can have sex with is not merely a matter of individual freedom and choice. In many cultures, same-sex relationships, for example, are not endorsed, and in many cases are not legal. Even what kinds of sex are possible is often a matter of legislation.

Foucault shows how this has not always been the case. In earlier times in western culture, for example in fifth-century Greece, sexual expression was governed in very different ways, openly allowing same-sex relationships, and even relationships between men and boys. In order to contrast the control of sexuality, Foucault shows how, for the ancient Greeks, regulating the appetite for food was much more of a concern. Within the Greek culture the regulation of food was a major priority, and individuals were expected to be moderate, reasoned and rational in food choice. Indeed, much was written about what foods could be eaten, when and with whom. Adherence to these forms of self-regulation was a sign that individuals could regulate their own appetites and, in so doing, could practise moderation and self-restraint, which is tantamount to reason. These characteristics were a prerequisite if one was to take part in decisions about the regulation of the city or the *polis*. While the need to be moderate was an individual consideration, there was support for it from within the culture. Immoderate activities, or hubris, although not punishable, were frowned on and denounced. In a later essay on the developments of these characteristics within a Christian context, Foucault shows how the admiration for moderation in the Greek and Roman cultures transforms to a requirement for asceticism and denial in the Christian tradition. Thus, in both eras, Greco-Roman and Christian, food regulation by the individual is highly regarded.

Restraint in a modern context

The contrast with current social and cultural norms could not be greater. In our modern secular world we are rewarded for wanting and consuming more, not less. There are no restraints on our appetites for food or indeed for other material possessions. And there are a number of consequences of this consumption.

One consequence is waste. In the area of food, for example, we witness a large amount of food being wasted. In Australia, something like $5 billon worth of food is wasted each year. In the UK the figure is about $16 billion. However, so rooted is our practice of wasting food that it simply goes unnoticed by most of us. For example, a recent study of household food waste in the UK carried out by the Waste and Resources Action Programme (WRAP) found that 90 per cent of the people polled claimed that they wasted little food – in many cases they said they wasted hardly any. Yet we know this not to be the case, and that most households waste alarming amounts of food. Thus there appears to be a disconnect between what people think they do and what they actually do. This is not good for promoting self-restraint, which requires a sense of awareness about what one eats, what one does not eat, and what one wastes. Without some form of self-reflection the possibilities of reining in food intake, as part of some lifestyle correction campaign, is going to be difficult.

The other consequence is excessive body fat. The rise in overweight people and obesity in most countries is the subject of much research, which we will not cover here. What is of more interest is the observation that rising levels of body fat are part of a changing picture of regulation. A number of scholars have traced the so-called 'obesity epidemic' to the time when many economies became deregulated and government regulation shrank. The transition to free-market economies in the 1980s, under what is known as neo-liberalism, is thought to have ramped up levels of consumption. Economically, this is of benefit. More consumption means, generally, more capital growth, greater spending, higher employment and other positive indicators of a healthy economy. Any regulation by government to restrain the market or temper growth is regarded to be unnecessary interference. In the eyes of many academics, the growth in the economy is matched by the growth in population girth. Boyd Swinburn and Gary Egger, in their book *Planet Obesity*, suggest that the obesity epidemic is but collateral damage resulting from unregulated consumerism – in other words, a consumptogenic environment.

Re-establishing food and regulation

Re-establishment of a culture of regulation is going to be hard work. This is why the healthy-eating campaigns discussed earlier are unable to deliver. All indicators are that, despite considerable effort by governments and other organisations charged with the responsibility of addressing rising levels of body weight, more and more adults and children are getting fatter. The need for governments to regulate a number of factors has never been greater. In an unrelated area, the necessity of this has become obvious.

The global financial crisis (GFC) developing from 2007 onwards is thought to be mostly due to a failure to regulate a number of financial and banking sectors. There is a belief that the crisis developed from a combined effect of: first, buyers desiring more than they could pay for in the housing market and over-extending themselves financially; second, a financial sector too willing to lend money to buyers whose overall capital position and long-term security was precarious; and finally, the subsequent ballooning of housing markets which became oversupplied, with a consequent decrease in market value of homes. When the market began to falter, home prices plummeted and selling up to pay for a mortgage was not an option. This scenario was played out in a number of economies from the US, to Ireland and the UK. Governments, such as Australia, that had regulated their banking systems to rein in excessive lending practices by banks were spared. The example proves that there is sense in having government regulation as a shield between the market and consumer.

Better food regulation – but how far does the public want government to go?

Thus there have been calls for governments to better regulate other systems where the consumers are unprotected from the free market, and where the current ethos is *caveat emptor*. In the area of food, this has concerned a range of issues, such as food marketing to children, labelling of food and extravagant claims about the healthiness of some food ingredients. Quite how far the public would like the government to go in regulating food is uncertain. Do we want to ban food companies from sponsoring children's sports? Would we welcome health warnings on food (such as *This food is high in sugar. Foods high in sugar could damage health if consumed in large amounts*)? How do we feel about putting a tax on foods that are high in fat (a so-called Fat Tax)?

And would any of this work, anyway? In answer to the last question, research in New Zealand suggests that taking the goods and services tax (GST) off a range of healthy foods would pay in the long run. Researchers demonstrated that removing the 15 per cent GST from a range of healthy foods – such as fresh fruit and vegetables, low-fat dairy foods, lean meats – led to a significant increase in sales in a group of randomly selected shoppers. The increased sales were much higher than those of another group of shoppers, which was only given information and advice about what is good to eat – in other words, current practice. Since the healthy foods are the foundations of the healthy diet that is supposed to lower chances of a range of chronic diseases, the long-term consequences for health, and for the overall economy, could be substantial. In summary, the research shows that government intervention to help people make healthy food choices can work. Self-restraint, without support, is highly unlikely, especially when excess and hubris are part of normal, everyday practice.

Closing remarks on food and regulation

The focus of regulation through the lens of food allows an examination of personal, political and international forces that are at play to shape and control our appetites. It has been the case that we have usually relied on governments to shield us from outside danger, and even from our own hubris. However, it is clear that government involvement in regulation has decreased, especially with modern economic models which warn against regulation of individuals, and assume that the market will sort things out. But it is hard to see how this is likely, given that self-restraint is difficult to control in the face of excess. Even harder is to find any time in human history when we have experienced the abundance of food at the same time as the lack of any barriers that assist us to control ourselves. The future does indeed look bleak.

Further reading

Coveney, J., In praise of hunger: Public health and the problem of excess. In *Mortality, Morbidity and Morality in the New Public Health*. edited by K. Bell and A. Salmon. New York: Routledge, 2011.

Egger, G. and Swinburn, B., *Planet Obesity: How We're Eating Ourselves and the Planet to Death*. St Leonards: Allen and Unwin, 2010.

Hamilton, C. and Denniss, R., *Affluenza: When Too Much is Never Enough*. St Leonards: Allen and Unwin, 2005.

6

FOOD AS ... THE ENVIRONMENT

Introduction

At the time of writing the Australian federal government has launched a report called the National Food Plan (NFP). According to the blurb, it is a call to action to ensure that the food supply in Australia is well positioned to take commercial opportunities, both at home and abroad, ensuring the food industry is competitive and fully optimised (for example, using the latest technology, skills and research) and that Australia is food secure, meaning that the population has available a food supply that is safe, affordable and nutritious. The NFP has come under fire from a number of quarters. The loudest protests have come from groups pointing out that a discussion of sustainability is conspicuous by its absence. It is argued that, while Australia produces enough food to feed 60 million people per year – well in excess of the needs of a nation population of about 25 million – the continued impact of the food supply on the environment has not been addressed in the NFP.

The debate highlights a concern that is now well developed in public discourse, which essentially boils down to the relationship between humans, the food supply and the environment. This debate's trajectory, which is part of the focus of this chapter, is interesting to follow. Thus we will look at how issues like sustainability and conserving a balance between humans and the environment come into focus when food is used as a lens.

Humans, food and the environment

It might be easy to think the impact of food on the environment is a relatively recent phenomenon. However, there is much evidence to demonstrate that food production by humans has always had a real or potential impact on our natural environment. It may appeal to our nostalgia to think back to times when humans were at one with nature. Yet the relationship between humans and their food supply, and the effects on the environment, have been precarious at best, and, at worse, highly environmentally damaging. This is not the place to examine in detail how, by producing food, humans damaged the environment, but some examples are needed. There is some agreement that the agriculture of cropping developed in regions we might call the Middle East – Iran and Iraq – over 5,000 years ago. These populations are now described at Sumerians, and they were successful at cultivating the wild grasses that were available in the region, like wheat and barley, into crops. The seeds could be sown, harvested and stored, thus reducing the need to constantly forage for food. The result was a regular supply of staple food. However, the success was not sustained. This was because poor irrigation practices upset a water–salt balance in the soil. Rising salt levels resulted, crop production gradually collapsed and the Sumerian population could not be sustained and had to migrate. In a very different location we have another example. The populations – now called Maori – that arrived in New Zealand from the Pacific Islands about 800 years ago are believed to have hunted the Moa, a large flightless bird, to extinction. Finally, there is evidence, controversial it has to be admitted, that the 'burning off' practices by Indigenous people in Australia – to flush out wildlife and stimulate growth of fire-dependent plants and produce new fruit and seeds – have been highly destructive for a number of plants and animals.

Of course, humans have managed to survive and adapt in these changed conditions, and it is true that the things learned have provided humans with better knowledge of growing and producing food. But that does not take away from the fact that the environment has been affected, sometimes permanently. One of the ways of surviving in the changed conditions is for human populations to shrink, or at least stagnate, so that there are fewer mouths to feed. This is part of a biological brake on population growth, because poor food intake produces malnutrition, which increases rates of morbidity and mortality; plus human fertility drops when food supplies are short. For long periods of history this biological balance between food, populations and survival was enough to sustain human development. However, there has been a slow growth in populations, even at times when food supplies have been short and more food has been required.

Population growth, food and the environment

The need to feed more people as populations grow is a concern that has a long history. Most famously this issue was addressed by Thomas Malthus in the eighteenth century. Malthus noted that as populations continue to grow, they will gradually outstrip their food supply. He predicted that eventually mass famine and disease would result. His predictions did not come to pass because of developments from the mid-nineteenth century that revolutionised the food supply. This happened at a number of levels. First, there was a major change in methods of crop production, arising mostly from the research of Justus von Leibig in Germany. Leibig and his group discovered that application of potassium, phosphate and nitrogen (as ammonia) to the soil accelerated growth of plants. The resulting mixture of KPN fertiliser created a major change in farming practices in North America and Europe. The result was a rise in wheat production and a fall in the price of staples such as bread (helped in England by the repealing of the Corn Laws in 1846, which allowed cheaper imported wheat from North America to flood the English market). The other development was the rise of a food industry that flourished with better transport of primary products, raw materials into factories and a better distribution to markets. The mass use of ice, and later refrigeration to keep food fresh, was also of great importance. Globalised food systems also played a role as Australia and New Zealand in Asia, and Argentina in South America, became providers of meat and dairy products to markets in Europe. The overall impact on the environment of these developments in the food supply was not great, simply because the scale of the change was relatively small. This was despite the fact that widespread and repeated applications of KPN fertilisers created noticeable deteriorations in soil health, a problem that was later addressed with better soil management and more sophisticated fertiliser formulations. The inputs into the food system – cheap raw materials and increasingly hi-tech machinery for processing – were all in plentiful supply. We saw in Chapter 4 that the food productionism paradigm in the post-Second World War period was able to ramp up food supplies to a staggering degree, creating a virtuous cycle in which increasingly available supplies of cheap food supported the growth of populations. Of course, this is not to say that there was a global benefit in these developments. Many countries in Africa and Asia experienced famines and food shortages. But even here, where possible, the excess food supplies from the wealthier countries were converted into food aid in times of shortage.

The shortage of oil and the food supply

A major event took place in the 1970s when the product that fuelled the food industry, and also so many other industries – oil – was short in supply. This is not the place to discuss why and how this happened: a number of excellent books have already been written on the subject. Here we might reflect on the impact of the oil shortage: food costs increased as oil in the form of gas or petrol became more costly; many of the applications in the primary production of foods were petroleum-based, and their availability was in question. Even though the global oil shortage lasted for only a couple of years, and things returned to nearly pre-oil shortage conditions shortly thereafter, the genie was now out of the bottle in the form of debates about an increasingly political topic: sustainability. Although countries such as the UK had to confront the sustainability of its food supply during the world wars it had engaged in during the first half of the twentieth century, this was mostly about a dependence on reliable sources of food. Now the issue was about dependence on reliable sources of fossil fuel, which was known to be in limited supply. Thus the industrial nature of the food supply, now known as *Big Food*, which was discussed in an earlier chapter, was increasingly called into question.

Industrialised environments and food

Other aspects of *Big Food* in the post-Second World War era were also causing alarm. Although food production was high, this was because of the industrialised nature of the system. There was a growing awareness of the impact of certain industrialised agricultural practices on the land and the soil. The development of KPN fertiliser has already been mentioned. However, the application of products like pesticides and herbicides was also being questioned. One of the milestones in this journey was the publication of Rachel Carson's *Silent Spring*, which critiqued the use of a number of applications which at the time were part of common agricultural practices. Chief among these was the use of DDT (dichlorodiphenyltrichloroethane). Carson's work confirmed that DDT is a powerful pesticide, but also that it has a lasting impact on various animal species because it leaves a residue in the land and the food supply. At the time the use of DDT – and other chemicals that did not break down over time to less harmful components – was widespread. They accumulated in the food supply, rising to toxic levels. Not only were these levels harmful to the environment, they were also suspected of causing harm to human health through developments of certain cancers.

Another example of attempts to grow more food via an intensive process is the so-called *Green Revolution*. Starting in Mexico and spreading to many other middle- to low-income countries, such as India, the Green Revolution was hailed as the answer to food production and to economic prosperity and stability for those countries that adopted it. As some have pointed out, however, while there have been increased crop yields, these have been at the expense of environmental damage due to crop overproduction.

The food supply and climate change

The last ten years have seen a further development in concerns about the impact of humans on the environment. This has been in the form of climatic changes, such as extreme weather events and rising global temperatures. The cause seems to be increasing levels of greenhouse gases – for example, carbon dioxide, nitrous oxide and methane. These gases can trap heat in the atmosphere. Increasing levels of greenhouse gases are thought to result from human activities: burning fossil fuels, removing carbon 'sinks' such as forests and trees, increasing levels of products that break down to nitrous oxide or methane.

There is a two-way relationship between the food supply and the factors that create climate change. This is because the food supply is substantially affected by climate change, yet it generates climate change precursors. For example, the food supply has been shown to be a significant contributor to the generation of greenhouse gases. This is through, first, the use of fossil fuels in applications used widely in food production, such as pesticides, herbicides and fertilisers. Fossil fuels are also used extensively in food industries, including transport and distribution. The primary production of food also creates large amounts of greenhouse gases, through, for example, the gases produced by ruminant animals – notably cattle and sheep – where large amounts of carbon dioxide and methane are belched up during the ruminant digestion processes. Methane is a particularly powerful green-house gas with an effect 20 times greater than carbon dioxide. Nitrogen-containing applications to crops – for example, fertili-sers – are also thought to contribute to greenhouse gases through microbial conversion to nitrous oxide, another potent green-house gas with an atmosphere warming effect of over 300 times more than carbon dioxide. Finally, waste in the food supply, much of which ends up in landfill, can ferment and produce methane. There are many other aspects of the food supply that impact on precursors of climate change. However, the relation-ship between the food supply and climate change also acts in the opposite direction: climate change influences the food supply. This is because rising temperatures affect crop production, espe-cially during long spells without rain. There is a belief that the Australian seven-year drought was a product of climate change resulting from human-induced greenhouse gas emissions. The drought had a major impact on food prices and the sustainability of many industries, especially those that relied on a plentiful supply of rainwater from river systems and other waterways, many of which were much reduced during the drought. The food supply is also affected by extreme weather events that might arise from climate change. In many parts of the world, soaring summer temperatures have created widespread bushfires that damage crops and endanger livestock, which interrupts the food supply. Also disruptive are the heavy rains and floods that are other aspects of extreme weather events. Cyclones, too, have had an enormous impact on food-producing parts of the world.

In Australia, while droughts have been part of the cyclic nature of the climate, drought events during the last ten years have had a massive impact on the food supply. One of the major food sources in Australia, the Murray Darling Basin, through which the rivers Murray, Darling and Murimbidgee flow, has seen significant changes in the kinds of foods grown and the use of water and other elements necessary for food production. Whole food sectors – citrus growers, wheat producers, livestock companies – have had to alter the ways in which their industries operate. For many, a scheme of water rationing – which was deemed necessary because of the effects of drought on the river systems from which water was removed to support food systems – has had a serious effect on business. More recently, extreme weather events such as floods and cyclones have removed whole commodities from the shop shelves. This has been most noticeable where it has affected fresh foods such as bananas, but other foods have also been affected. The predictions of increased ambient temperatures, if realised, will also have an effect on food production. Some areas that have been traditional food sources might become too dry, salty and hot.

Food and the ocean environment

The impact of the food supply on the ocean has been one of the most dramatic examples of how we can understand changing environments through the food lens. Arguably, for millennia the sea and ocean environments have provided food supplies for human populations. This food has been in the form of fish, shellfish, sea mammals (whales), sea plants and so on. Populations have come to depend on these sources of food, and it is also the case that some animal life, such as birds, have benefited from human involvement in ocean food supplies. These synergistic relationships are common in the human–food–environment triangle. However, in some parts of the world the supply of fish stocks has fallen. One of the most dramatic events was the collapse of the cod industry on the east coast of Canada, in parts of the UK and in Scandinavia. The potential problems of 'overfishing' had been sounded for many years, and the evidence of falling fish stocks was in the dwindling number of fish catches. There are warnings that overfishing in other parts of the world – for example, the Southern Ocean's tuna stocks – is possible. Indeed, one prediction is that by 2050 all commercial fishing will have ceased because of overfishing practices. Much of the problem lies with the large-scale nature of fishing boats, where nets the size of football pitches trawl the ocean and engulf large numbers of fish. These volumes of catch do not allow adequate time for replenishment and renewal of fish stocks. Thus, many fish species are in danger. This is having an effect further up the food chain as consumers are more aware of what wise seafood purchases might be.

Overfishing has also given rise to fish farming, a practice that has been part of some cultures – especially in Asia – for thousands of years. One of the most common fish farming products is Atlantic salmon, which has become a dominant product in the marketplace. The practice of fish farming varies, but a common method is to net off a part of the ocean shore and rear the salmon from fingerlings. However, because they are not free to forage for food, the salmon needs to be provided with stocks of food in the form of fishmeal. The meal has to be brought from elsewhere, and there have been some concerns about the quality and safety of this product. Some viruses, for example, have been found to reside in the meal and this affects the eventual quality of the salmon. Another problem is the waste that arises from the closed environment in which the salmon are reared. Lacking an adequate flushing and refreshing of the pen in which they are raised, the fish are in danger of growing in cramped and unsanitary conditions.

Public reaction to food and the environment

Having looked at a number of environmental issues that arise when the lens of food is used, we should consider how in the name of better food a number of groups are developed with the view of improving the food supply. The work of Rachel Carson, mentioned earlier, was extremely important in increasing awareness of the impact of the food supply on environmental and human health. Carson's findings gave impetus to a movement that was increasingly opposed to the industrialised nature of agriculture, questioning the safety of many products that were commonly used at the time. We would now recognise this as the growing organic industry, or more particularly the permaculture movement. Parallel to this was another movement that was raising consciousness and developing what might be regarded as a consumer movement. The work by US campaigner Ralph Nader also had a particular focus on safety and sustainability of the food supply. Nader's campaigning raised many questions about the safety of many additives used in the food supply: whether these were colourings, flavourings, preservatives or manufacturing agents (gels, anti-caking agents, etc.). Overall, the major concerns were that industrialisation of food production and food manufacturing and processing were a danger to human and environmental health.

By the early 1960s, in places like the US and Europe there were a number of well-developed groups that were lobbying for changes to the food supply so that it was less industrialised and more in tune with natural processes that would benefit humans and the environment. These groups – like Friends of the Earth and Greenpeace – provided information for government and the public about what the consequences were of the rapidly developing food system, which had many features that were worrying from an environmental perspective. One of the most recent examples of the work of these groups has been the engagement with the development of genetically modified organisms (GMO) and their use in the food supply. During the latter part of the twentieth century, a number of biotechnological developments provided the opportunity to produce new kinds of crops. Note that new crop varieties and hybrids are common in modern agronomic science. These are usually developed for higher yields, greater resistance to pests, easier cropping, and so on. Advances in biotechnology allowed for the development of new types of crops that had spliced into their DNA genes that conferred new properties to the plants. The important point here is that the added genes were not always from other plants, as is the case with conventional hybridisation or cross-fertilisation. The genes were from other life forms, such as bacteria. The results were crops with characteristics that had never been developed before. Some crops have genes from the *Bacillus thuringiensis* (BT) bacteria. The overall effect of the BT gene is to confer to the crop a toxic effect to grubs, caterpillars and similar pests. Another gene has been engineered into plants to make them immune to the effects of a herbicide called Roundup. The resulting plants are called Roundup Ready. When Roundup is applied to crops the Roundup Ready plants are resistant and are spaced, while weeds and other plant life are destroyed.

The potential for these biotechnology developments to do good in improving the yield of crops, reduce damage from herbicide and pesticide applications that are currently in use and essentially advance benefits to humankind, goes without saying. However, there has been widespread public and government concern about the safety of these products, which are now in use in many countries, especially in North and South America. Questions arise as to the environmental effects, especially to local animal and plant life which shares the same habitat. Cross-contamination – or 'outcropping', where genes from the GMO crop transfer to other crops (which could be weeds which would themselves become herbicide resistant) – has also been a concern. Other groups have raised worries about the safety of GMOs to humans, asking questions about the nature and the integrity of the safety testing procedures.

These examples provide a clear picture of how food provides ways in which people have rallied around a cause. Environmental concerns have also had an impact on what people are choosing to eat, and other food practices. For example, a number of local government authorities are campaigning to reduce household food waste to reduce environmental impacts, but also address what is called 'waste in vain': that is, food which has embodied waste by virtue of it being invested with energy (mostly from fossil fuel) as part of its production. Efforts to address sustainability of the food supply go back as far as 1996 when sustainable dietary guidelines were suggested. One of the major features of these guidelines is a reduction in the amount of meat from ruminants. Eating further down the food chain, by incorporating more plant-based foods such as fruits and vegetables is another priority. As well as the type of food, the origin of the food and its journey from the producer to the consumer is also considered to be important. However, each country, and even regions within countries, will need to make their own recommendations. For example, from where I write (Adelaide, Australia), a diet with locally sourced foods such as chicken and eggs, wheat-based products and fresh fruits and vegetables would be entirely suitable. Even wine would be sustainable because of proximity to local vineyards. In another country, say, in northern Europe, different recommendations would need to be made to suit the local environment.

Closing remarks about food as environment

The need for food has meant that humans have had to interact with their environment. As we have seen, this relationship has not always been sustainable. History tells us that when human populations have not been able to employ agricultural methods that are not compatible with the cycles and rhythms of nature, then the results can be catastrophic. For a large part of human history, any environmental disasters could be overcome by population migration to pastures new. With increased settlement and population expansion, this is not always possible. Thus the pressure on the land to produce more food is intense. Whether technology will be able to rescue humans from the problems we now face is hard to say. Some of the solutions appear to add to the problem, as we have seen. However, what is clear is the engagement with the problem by community groups and like-minded citizens. Eating low on the food chain is a possible way of addressing the problems of environmental degradation and climate change. However, the extent to which this is possible for large numbers of the population is uncertain. Also uncertain is whether a more environmentally friendly food supply is even seen to be desirable in populations in growing economies that are enjoying the kind of lifestyle that westerners have been used to for some years. What is certain is that the current environmental impact of food production and food consumption is contributing to the issues of food justice – who gets to eat what. This is the subject of the next chapter.

Further reading

Friel, S. and Dangour, A., *et al.*, Impact on public health of strategies to reduce greenhouse gas emissions: food and culture. *Lancet* 374, 2016–25, 2009.

Lang, T., Barling, D. and Caraher, M., *Food Policy: Integrating Health, Environment and Society.* Oxford: Oxford University Press, 2009.

Stuart, T., *Waste: Uncovering the Global Food Scandal*, New York: W.W. Norton, 2009.

7

FOOD AS ... JUSTICE

Introduction

In earlier chapters we looked at the question of who eats what. We examined this in terms of social issues, such as the ways in which someone's social class demarcates what is eaten, and we looked at cultural determinants – in other words, the ways in which different cultural groups draw on what is available to be called 'food' and mark that out as cultural territory or boundaries. Food is often used to stereotype various cultures, and is often shorthand for what a culture might be described to be. Other chapters highlighted the role of food as identity, pointing out that what we eat is a powerful marker to others, and indeed ourselves, about who we are.

In this chapter, instead of examining who eats what, we will look at the question of 'Who gets what to eat?'. This question sets up a powerful argument for food as justice. Justice allows a view of food access and availability that brings into focus a number of important considerations. For example, there is a lively conversation about the way 'Who gets what to eat?' is actually a human rights question. In other words, there is an agreement that having enough food to eat is a fundamental human right.

Asking the question 'Who gets what to eat?' also highlights some examples of the unfair ways in which some populations are ignored yet some are privileged in terms of food availability. Food justice – as it is often called – also highlights the ways in which some populations are not able to control their food destiny. For example, when new technologies are introduced, traditional food production methods can be marginalised or even forgotten, leaving the food supply in the hands of the few who do not represent the majority. Finally, embedded in the question 'Who gets what to eat?' is another question, and that is 'and how much do they get?'. Thus, food as justice allows us to look at questions of food quantity and also food quality. We will look at these issues in turn.

Food justice, a short political history

The centrality of food in human development is a major theme in this book. We need food to develop human cultural and social patterns. We need food to establish and maintain our identities. But the most important aspect in our lives is the need for food to survive. Indeed, the basic necessity of food for survival has, arguably, been at the centre of human development, and indeed, political change. In his book *The Politics of Provision*, John Bohstedt points to the way that food shortages in England from the sixteenth to the nineteenth century transformed that country's political and governmental processes. At times of food shortage, when crops failed through drought or pestilence, whole populations rioted and took the law – some would say justice – into their own hands. Brute force to quell rioters was a poor solution to the problem and the longer-term

proposition of providing food relief was seen to be more attractive. England moved from a hand-to-mouth agrarian culture to a
mixed economy where the widespread trading of food became a
feature of English commerce in the eighteenth and nineteenth
centuries. This was helped no doubt by the colonies which
clothed and fed the growing English population. In another
setting, the nineteenth century Irish potato famine – and the
injustice to that failed to redistribute food to the starving – was
central to the Irish diaspora which led to a mass movement of the
Irish population to North America and Australia. The result was
a transformation of social and political life in those places. And let
us not forget that the shortage of wheat for bread-making was
one of the precipitating factors that is said to have caused the
French Revolution. Whether or not the king's wife, Marie
Antoinette, actually said 'Let them eat cake' – or more probably
brioche, a cake-like bread – is a moot point. But if even a myth,
it was indicative of the indifference of the French Court to the
plight of the French peasants, who were starving because of food
shortage. Again, the consequences of this food injustice was
major – leading to a new form of French governance based on
the republic, or people rule. We can see therefore that
food-related injustices have been central to social, political and
economic transformations, and have, and will continue to have,
major effects on human development.

Rights-based approaches to food justice

The right of people to have access to enough food was enshrined
in the Universal Declaration of Human Rights when these
were first drafted after the Second World War. As we have
seen, the expectation that people would have enough to eat
was at the heart of many social and political movements
before that. However, the visibility of food as a basic right for
people was a milestone in international political history. The

right to have enough food puts an obligation on authorities, such as governments, to ensure that the people they serve are adequately fed.

This development has been something new. It was not unusual for many governments, especially in developing countries, to expect that some people would simply go without food. Indeed, feeding the world's population, which is believed to be ever increasing, has been an ongoing political and economic consideration ever since Thomas Malthus proposed the idea that growing populations would eventually outstrip the supply of food available to them. Thus famines, droughts and food shortages became things to endure – and even expect – as part of the way of life in some countries. The fact that there is not enough food to go around was an expectation and a frequent experience.

However, there has been a growing realisation that there is in fact enough food in the world to feed everyone adequately. That is to say, we now know that annual global food production is sufficient to feed every woman, man and child on the planet. Thus the question of why some people do not get enough to eat becomes a question of why is it that food is not distributed evenly or fairly across the world. Why do some countries have more, and some have less?

Food justice and human disaster

It is true that human crises or disasters are often the cause of food mal-distribution. Many food shortages are caused by mass movement of populations from their homes, and therefore from reliable food supplies, because of threats of war or other fears for human safety. At the time of writing, news is spreading of mass movement of people from their homes in the People's Republic of Congo, where ongoing fighting between pro- and anti-government armies has displaced civilians. When people are at a distance from their own food supplies they have to be fed from emergency or relief supplies, which are often shipped into refugee camps or other places of temporary settlement. A vivid picture of what food injustice looks like for families in this situation can be found in the book *The Hungry Planet: What the World Eats* by photographer Peter Menzel and writer Faith D'Aluisio. Essentially the book documents what food and drink is consumed over a week by 30 families from 24 countries around the globe, taking in the developed and developing worlds. One of the families is in the Darfur region of Sudan. The family are refugees and their meagre week's worth of food is laid out on the ground outside their makeshift home or tent. The food comprises rations of cereals like sorghum and something called corn–soy blend, donated by the World Food Programme. Water and fuel for cooking also have to be rationed. The fate of this family represents the state of affairs for all the families in this refugee camp, and indeed families in other camps housing refugees or where military activity affects civilians.

One of the long-term consequences of population displace-ment such as this is that even if and when food supplies are re-established, it is often the case that the experience of being dependent on donor countries for food is enduring. Thus the move back to self-sufficiency is often difficult. Food justice often implies another term; that of food security. Here we will under-stand food security to mean that individuals, communities and populations have control over what foods they have access to and under what terms and conditions.

While food security often invokes discussions about what food sources are available to people in countries where food supplies are precarious or unreliable, we might also apply the term to communities in so-called advanced economies. For although the supply of food appears to be adequate, even excessive, in places like Australia, the US, UK and other similar jurisdictions, the extent to which people have control over what is offered for sale is often questionable. The notion of food 'choice' is often used to indicate the way that people living in relatively rich economies are able to select foods from a wide variety. However, it can be argued that on closer inspection there are often few real 'choices'. Instead, what is happening is what is called 'choice editing'. This process is undertaken within each supermarket chain or similar retailer, where decisions are made about what will be offered for sale. These decisions are made with regard to supply, demand, profit, throughput, etc. And what is offered is not always what people actually want, or what might be healthy for them. The mainstream food supply is dominated mostly by processed and other foods that have been selected by the retailer. Of course, supermarkets offer fresh foods and so-called healthy alternatives. However, a look down the aisle with breakfast cereals – or worse, biscuits and snacks – tells all. Mostly what is offered is similar in composition, and often with unhealthy ingredients. There are often alternatives, such as 'whole foods', 'organic foods' or 'fair trade', but these are often few in number and often more expensive. Thus the idea that customers 'choose' foods is somewhat misleading and many people are rightfully suspicious of the idea that we have real choice and food justice. Also regarded as suspicious is the idea that consumers should be required to choose foods from the vast array of what is on offer; food marketing is highly sophisticated and foods are often promoted on dubious grounds. For example, healthy benefit claims might be downright misleading, and yet consumers are required to make informed choices even when the facts are doubtful. So while the idea of food security grew and developed in less affluent countries, where traditional foodways are being eroded, questions of control of food provenance or destiny in more well-off countries need to be asked. Indeed, the idea of knowing where food actually comes from – its provenance – is increasingly problematic. It is to this area that we now turn.

Food justice and food technology

The precarious nature of control over food destiny is never so visible as in the case of populations where new technologies have been introduced with the promise of increasing food supply. Building on the belief that world food supplies are shrinking in the face of rapidly rising populations, a number of initiatives have been introduced to developing countries. One of the most famous, mentioned in an earlier chapter, was the so-called *Green Revolution* developed during the 1960s and 1970s.

The 'revolution' was based on the development of hybrid strains of staple foods like corn and rice. The application of high levels of fertiliser and other growth enhancements were found to increase yields beyond those of more traditional methods of crop production. During the 1970s a number of countries embraced the new forms of crop production, and indeed saw yields increase. However, the technology required to maintain the system – the hybrid seeds, the fertilisers and other applications – became an increasing financial burden for traditional farmers who had converted to the *Green Revolution*. Moreover, the new food system moved control from the farmers to the suppliers of the various new technologies. Thus actual food ownership shifted. Many countries, such as India, are still working out how to manage the eventual economy and other developments of the *Green Revolution*. There have been enormous social and cultural consequences which sees fewer people on the land – and thus a reduction of employment in a country that has traditionally seen farming as a main source of income for rural economies – and a disruption of the distribution chain from producers to consumers.

A similar scenario has been predicted with the introduction of genetically modified seeds. These are promoted on the basis of better yields without the need for frequent applications of pesticides or herbicides. The genetically modified seeds produce crops that have been engineered to either withstand the effects of applications of herbicides or to contain properties that are poisonous to insects. Their inbuilt toxicity or immunity to pests or herbicides is hailed as a major development in agriculture. However, unlike traditional methods of crop production where seeds from one year's crop are used to plant the next year's harvest, the genetically modified seeds have to be purchased every year, thus ensuring repeated purchases of seeds by producers on an annual basis. There are other ways in which food producers are mortgaged to the industries that promote these new technologies in food production. The point is that the technology does not release farmers, but instead binds them to the businesses that promote the new ways of food production. In doing so the actual control of the food supply changes, and the independence of food producers, and indeed the whole food chain, is changed.

Food justice and trade

Other ways in which food injustices are created can be seen from examples in which land used for food production has been used to grow other commodities. Why would this happen? More developed economies and trading blocs, like the US and the European Union, grow much more food than their populations can consume. The overproduction is often supported by government grants and subsidies. Effectively, this allows cheap food onto the world market. For poorer countries, which cannot support or subsidise food production, local foods are more expensive to produce. So home-grown staples are replaced by imported supplies. These changes are often part of the conditions that are imposed as part of economic packages offered to low-income countries. In these circumstances food production switches to production of other commodities, such as coffee, cut flowers or salad vegetables, which are exported onto a global market. The income from these exports is then used by locals to purchase the cheaper food imports. Whether this makes economic sense is debatable, but not debatable is the shift from self-sufficiency and food security, to food insecurity and precarious food sustainability. Left to the global markets, poorer countries now have to cope with fluctuations in global food prices. The price of food staples on the world market can change because of a number of reasons. For example, at the time of writing, massive droughts across the US have dramatically reduced the yield of corn, wheat and other crops. The US has been a major source of these crops on the world market. However, a major crisis is predicted because the supplies from the US will be limited due to the climate effects. Other reasons for fluctuations of world food prices might be the diversion of food crops into non-food industries. For example, the recent production of bio-fuels in the US has shunted large amounts of corn from the food supply to the production of ethanol as a fossil fuel substitute.

Rises in global food prices – which have been seen at times throughout the early part of the twenty-first century – have meant food shortages for those countries that have moved away from local food production to depend on food imports. It is not easy for producers to make the switch from a non-food crop back to a staple at these times to overcome costs of imported foods. Thus the injustices that accrue from exposure to the world food market become highly apparent. But food justice is not only about food quantity. Food quality is also a justice issue, as is explained in the next section.

Food justice and food quality

The distribution of foods of poor quality is a major economic and health problem for many countries. Many examples exist of poor-quality food being sold off by one country to a poor neighbour. One of the best examples is where the butchering of livestock in big livestock-producing countries such as Australia and New Zealand produces high levels of low-quality cuts of meat, which are sometimes used for animal consumption via pet food production. However, these cuts are often exported to developing countries. For example, 'mutton flaps', which are cuts of meat from the rib area of mature sheep, are exported to countries in the Pacific, such as Fiji, Tonga and Samoa. In the meat industries in Australia and New Zealand the flaps are considered difficult cuts from which to trim lean meat, and are not cost effective to process. So they are frozen for sale off-shore. These cuts have become entrenched in the diets of many Pacific Island populations, where they have displaced more traditional foods. Not only are they unhealthy for humans – mutton flaps are high in fat – they are also unhealthy for the economy because they undercut what can be produced locally. A similar example exists for what are called 'turkey tails'. These are off-cuts from the turkey-processing industry, mainly in the US. Turkey tails are extremely high in fat, and are sold off to many poorer countries in the Pacific region. The price and popularity of these fatty ends of turkey have made them popular with some Pacific Island populations. However, the consequences for public health have been disastrous. So much so that one country, Samoa, imposed a ban on importation of turkey tails in an effort to reduce the availability of this highly fatty food, which was considered to be a major contributor to levels of overweight and obesity. However, the ban had to be lifted as a condition for Samoa to become a member of the World Trade Organization. One of the long-term consequences of mass availability of cheap foods, such as turkey tails and mutton flaps, is that reliance on these eventually erodes knowledge and practices of local food production. Thus a vicious cycle of dependency is established.

Re-establishing food justice

The need to increase justice in the food supply is a hotly debated issue. This is not only needed for countries where food transitions are happening, such as in the developing world, but also in more developed economies. Indeed, in the latter we can see a number of initiatives that are designed to give people more control over their food. Some of these have already been discussed in earlier chapters. For example, the establishment of alternative food systems such as farmers' markets, organic schemes, community gardens and other non-conventional sources of food can count as ways in which some people are trying to regain control and exercise justice – however small that might be – over their food supply.

Indeed, there is a belief that consumers are not as powerless as they might think. While alternative food systems are very much in the minority compared to the size and power of the large supermarket chains or other conglomerates, they can give consumers an opportunity to regain control of their food supply. While for many people these systems are still very much complementary to the mainstream food supply, the fact that empowerment does occasionally exist is a form of emancipation that many people acknowledge. Even the smallest household, it is believed, can grow some edible plant for home consumption. And the support for this kind of home enterprise has exploded over recent years. In countries like Australia, sales of seeds and seedlings for food plants has sky-rocketed. As mentioned earlier, local government councils are establishing community gardens and other urban areas where people can grow and swap food. However, we run into the problem of justice even here. This is because most of these schemes are unlikely to attract low-income families unless they are well promoted and specifically targeted. It would seem that the idea of food justice is not evenly distributed across the social spectrum.

Food justice and food sovereignty

Beyond developed countries we can see examples of movements that are trying to establish what is known as 'food sovereignty'.

Indeed, the term 'food sovereignty' was first used with what is known as the Via Campesina movement, also known as the 'Peasants' Way'. This worldwide network is used to promote control over food provenance and food destiny. It grew out of a number of smaller initiatives that recognised that farmers and small food producers were losing land to larger corporations and multinationals. Foundational issues for the movement are that the heart of the food system should be those people who produce, distribute and consume food, and not large corporations and free markets; and that the land, water, seeds, and biodiversity necessary to produce a food supply needed to nourish individuals and communities should rest with the people themselves. Also embedded in the foundational understandings within Via Campesina is the notion with which we start this chapter – that of food being a human right.

This is echoed in the Food Sovereignty movement in Australia and the Australian Food Sovereignty Alliance. As with Via Campesina, the Alliance grew out of grassroots concerns that rural communities generally and food producers in particular were becoming more vulnerable to large corporate concerns. For example, a number of local, rural food economies in Australia have been reduced in size or even deleted as food companies have sought to move operations outside Australia. While the importation of food has long been part of the food system in many countries, especially those with shrinking food production sectors, such as the UK, the transition to the importation of food in a country like Australia is entirely new. Indeed, it is through this development that the agenda of movements like the Australian Food Sovereignty Alliance, and even the wider networks like Via Campesina, are being recognised. Australian consumers are not comfortable with food coming from other countries, since Australia has traditionally been a food producer and exporter. Other concerns about food safety when food is imported are also high on the agenda.

Closing remarks on food as justice

Food as justice provides a powerful lens through which to examine a number of contemporary as well as historical developments. The injustices associated with unfair food distribution have created a number of crises that have had major consequences for economic, social and political change. Some of these injustices are still with us, and, as we have seen in this chapter, poorer countries do not always fare well in the face of powerful, often globalised forces that dictate their food destiny. But food injustice is not only a developing country problem. As we have seen, even in so-called rich countries, food injustices are common and actions to address them are necessary.

Further reading

Bohstedt, J., *The Politics of Provisions: Food Riots, Moral Economy, and Market Transitions in England c.1550–1850*. Burlington, VT: Ashgate, 2010.

Huntley, R., *Eating Between the Lines: Food and Equity in Australia*. Victoria: Black Inc., 2008.

Jaffe, J. and Gertler, M., Victual vicissitudes: consumer deskilling and the (gendered) transformation of food systems. *Agriculture and Human Values* 23, 143–62, 2006.

Menzel, P. and D'Aluisio, F., *The Hungry Planet: What the World Eats*. Berkeley, CA: Ten Speed Press, 2005.

REFERENCES

Ten books that have informed and influenced my understanding of food and eating are listed here.

David, Elizabeth, *French Provincial Cooking*. London: Michael Joseph, 1965.

DeVault, Margorie, *Feeding the Family: The Social Organisation of Caring as Gendered Work*. Chicago, IL: University of Chicago Press, 1991.

Dixon, Jane, *The Changing Chicken: Chooks, Cooks, and Culinary Culture*. Sydney: UNSW Press, 2002.

Dye-Gussow, Joan, *Chicken Little, Tomato Sauce and Agriculture: Who Will Produce Tomorrow's Food?* New York: Bootstrap Press, 1991.

Grigson, Jane, *Good Things*. London: Michael Joseph, 1971.

Lang, Tim and Heasman, Michael, *Food Wars: The Global Battle for Mouths, Minds and Markets*. London: Earthscan, 2004.

McGee, Harold, *On Food and Cooking: The Science and Lore of the Kitchen*. New York: Scribner, 2004.

Moore Lappe, Frances, *Diet for a Small Planet*. New York: Friends of the Earth, 1971.

Symons, Michael, *One Continuous Picnic*. Adelaide: Duck Press, 1982.

Tallis, Raymond, *Hunger*. Stockfield: Acumen Publishing, 2008.

INDEX

access: history 88–9; and human
    rights 87–8, 89–90
additives 82
advertising 35, 49, 54, 58
affluence 35–6; and health 65–6;
    regulation of 65–8; rise in 64
Affluenza 67
affordability 1. *see also* prices
aging 23–4
agriculture: industrialisation 77–8;
    non-food crops 94–5; organic 82;
    origins 74; overproduction. 78
Albala, Ken, *Eating Right in the
    Renaissance* 10
allotments 42
alternative food systems 57–8, 97
anatomy 7
animal growth promoters 48
Annang community, the 22
anthropology 16–7
appetite, self-regulation 64–5
artisanal revival 47
Assize on Bread (1266) 62
Atwater, Wilbur 38–9, 40
Australia: artisanal revival 47;
    cooking skills 37–8; drought
    79–80; food contamination 62;
    food politics 33–4, 35; food
    production 73; Food Sovereignty
    movement 98; household
    expenditure 23; kitchen gardens

43; meat industry 95–6; milk price
    wars 52; National Food Plan
    (NFP) 73
Australian Food Sovereignty
    Alliance 98
authority 32
availability 1

Bacillus thuringiensis (BT) bacteria 83
basic necessity, the 88
behavioural psychology, and food
    choice 13, 15–7
belonging 19
Big Food 4, 41, 57; and the consumer
    52; definition 47, 50–1;
    development of 47–50;
    environmental impact 77, 77–8;
    food consumptionism 49–50; food
    productionism 48–9, 50; health
    impacts 53–6; industrialisation
    48–9, 82; intensification 48–9;
    and prices 51, 51–2; retail sector
    51; scale 51–3
Big Mac eaters 30
biochemistry 7
biodiversity 98
biofuels 95
biological adaptation 15–6
biotechnological developments
    83–4, 93–4
bodily renewal 20–1

body image, and identity 21–3
body size: and identity 21–3; and social networks 27
Bohstedt, John, *The Politics of Provision* 88–9
bones 20–1
Booth, Charles 16
Bordo, Susan 16
Bourdieu, Pierre 25–6; *Distinctions: A Social Critique of the Judgement of Taste* 16
bovine spongiform encephalopathy (BSE or 'mad cow disease') 62
box schemes 57
Bread Act (UK 1822) 62
BSE (bovine spongiform encephalopathy or 'mad cow disease') 62
Buddhism 63
burning off 75

Canada 81
cancer 78
cardiovascular diseases 65
Carson, Rachel, *Silent Spring* 78, 82
cattle, greenhouse gas emissions 79
celebrity chefs 58
cells and cellular development 7, 20–1
cellular damage 24
character 8
childhood obesity 55
children: advertising and 35; food market 34–5; and food politics 33–4, 34–6; fresh food and 57–8; obesity 55; pester power 35; roles 36; ultra-processed foods and 55
China, food contamination 62
choice editing 92
Christianity 28–9, 63, 68
class 16, 25–6
climate change 4, 78–80, 85
cod industry 81
colourings 48, 55
commodification 45
community, food politics 41–2

community gardens 97
community supported agriculture (CSA) 42–3
complexion 9
Congo, People's Republic of 90–1
conspicuous consumption 25
consumer, the, and Big Food 52
consumerism 69
consumption 49–50, 58, 68–9; conspicuous 25
consumptogenic environments 49–50, 66, 67, 69
consumptogensis 66
contamination 61–2
control 32
convenience foods 65
cooking 17; definition 37; education 37–8, 39; politics of 36–9; and ultra-processed foods 54, 55
cooking skills, decline in 36–8, 40–1, 54, 55
Corn Laws 76
cost of living 38–9
counter culture 41
crop yields 78
Crotty, Pat 13, 19–20
Culinary Triangle, the 17
cultural capital 25–6
cultural identity 13, 19–20, 29–30
culture: food as 16–7; and food choice 15–7

D'Aluisio, Faith 91
Darfur region 91
Davis, Clara 14–5
DDT (dichlorodiphenyltrichloroethane) 78
Denniss, Richard 67
dependency 96
diet: and aging 24; and humoral theory 11–2
dietary laws 28–9, 63–4, 66–7
dietary guidelines, sustainable 84
dietary lifestyle diseases 65–6

dietetic–gastronomic understanding 12–3
dietetics 7, 7–8; and humoral balance 9–13; role 10
Distinctions: A Social Critique of the Judgement of Taste (Bourdieu) 16
Dixon, Jane 49, 57
domestic science 39
drought 79–80, 90

Easter 66–7
eating disorders 16
eating healthy 26–7; campaigns 69
eating properly, and identity 28–9
Eating Right in the Renaissance (Abala) 10
education, cooking 37–8, 39
Egger, Gary 69
empirico-transcendental doublet, the 10–1
England, food shortages 88–9
environmental degradation 85
environmental impact 4–5, 73–85; *Big Food* 77, 77–8; biotechnological developments 84; burning off 75; climate change 78–80; drought 79–80; extinctions 75; fish stock decline 80–2; historical 74–5, 85; the ocean 80–2; overproduction. 78; population growth 75, 75–6; public reaction 82–4
everyday life, management of 7–8
exports 94–5, 96
exterior identity 20–1, 21–3
extinctions 75

family, the 4; children's roles 36; decision-making process 34; food industry impact on 56; micro-politics 32–3, 33–9; power in 34, 36
famine 21, 76, 90
farmers' markets 41–2, 57, 97
fast-food 50–1
fasting 66–7

fat 55
fatness 22–3, 69
feminism 33
fertilisers 48, 76, 77–8, 79, 93
Fischler, Claude 15
fish farming 81–2
fish meal 81
fish stocks 4, 80–2
fishing boats 81
flavour 55
flavourings 48
food aid 76, 91
food calibration methods 38–9
food choices 13–7, 26, 27, 92; behavioural 13, 15–7; innate 13–5
food chores 33
food consumptionism 49–50
food cultures 8, 16–7, 29–30
food defilement 61
food democracy 43, 97
food gardens 57–8
food identity 30
food industry 4, 32, 45–58; alternative food systems 57–8, 97; artisan 47; consumers 46; consumptionism 49–50; control 88; development of *Big Food* 47–50; globalisation 50–1; health impacts 53–6; impact on the family 56; industrialisation 48–9; intensification 48–9; issues 56–8; market driver 57; monopolies 52; producers 45–7; productionism 48–9, 50; retail sector 51, 57; scale 51–3; specialisations 47
food injustice 91, 99; consequences of 88–9
food justice 87–99; and choice 92; and food sovereignty 97–8; and food technology 93–4; history 88–9; and human disaster 90–2; and human rights 88, 89–90, 98; and quality 95–6; re-establishing 96–7; and trade 94–5
food knowledge 12
food market 45; segmentation 34–5

food miles 42, 84
food movements 41
food needs calculation 38–9
food origins 43, 46, 92, 98
food personalities 30
food plants, seed sales 97
food politics 32–44; advertising and
  35; and children 33–4, 34–6; and
  children's roles 36; community
  41–2; community supported
  agriculture (CSA) 42–3; of
  cooking 36–9; definition 32;
  family micro-politics 32, 33–9;
  and national security 39–41; pester
  power 35
food preparation skills, decline in
  37–8
food preservation 48, 76
food processing industry 53–6
food production: environmental
  impact 4–5, 73–85; knowledge 5
food productionism 48–9,
  50, 76
food quality: and food justice 95–6;
  legislation 61–3
food regulation, legislation 61–3
food security 39–41, 48, 91–3, 95
food shortages 88–9, 90
food sovereignty 93, 97–8
Food Sovereignty movement 98
food supply: control 46, 88; rural
  47–8; urban 47
food swaps 57, 97
food systems: alternative 57–8, 96–7;
  globalised 76
food technology, and food justice
  93–4
food-based movements 4, 98
Foucault, Michel: *History of Sexuality*
  67–8; *The Order of Things* 10–1
Framingham 27
France, regional foods 47
Fred the Foodie 1–2
free choice 15
free-market economies 69
French Revolution 89

fresh food 42–3, 53, 55–6; box
  schemes 57; children and 57–8;
  and climate change 80; markets
  46; prices 51, 56; shelf life 56;
  supermarket stocks 92;
  sustainability 85; taxation 71; and
  ultra-processed foods 55–6
Friends of the Earth 83
fruits 55
fuel 91; prices 77

Galen of Pergamum 8
garden schemes, schools 57–8
gardening 43, 57–8
Garibaldi metwurst (cooked
  sausage) 62
gastronomies 8
gastronomy 12–3
genetic modification 83–4, 93–4
Georgia 24
global financial crisis (GFC) 70
global warming 78–80
globalisation 30, 50–1, 76
GM crops 83–4, 93–4
goods and services tax (GST) 71
gout 23
government 32, 60, 63, 70–1, 71
Greece, ancient 10, 28, 67–8
Green Revolution, the 78, 93
greenhouse gas emissions 5, 46,
  78–80
Greenpeace 83
growth 3, 7

Hamilton, Clive 67
health 8; and food justice 95–6; and
  humoral balance 9–13; humoral
  theory 8–9; identity 26–7;
  legislation 66; and lifestyle 65–6;
  pesticides and 78; the role of
  dietetics 10; warnings 70–1
health identity 26–7
health warnings 70–1
healthism 29
healthy eating 29; campaigns 69
Heasman, M. 48

herbicides 48, 77–8, 79, 83, 84
Hinduism 63, 66
Hippocrates 8
History of Sexuality (Foucault) 67–8
home economics 37–8, 39
home science 39
home-cooked food 36–7
household expenditure 23, 64
human development 3, 6–18; central
    role of food 6–7; and cooking 17;
    dietetics 7, 7–8, 9–13; and food
    choice 13–7; and food knowledge
    13; social 4; understanding 6–7
human disaster, and food justice
    90–2
human rights, and food justice 88,
    89–90, 98
humors, the 8–9; balancing 9–13
*Hungry Planet: What the World Eats,
    The* (Menzel and D'Aluisio) 91
hypermarkets 51

identity 4, 19–30; and body image
    21–3; communicating 24–6;
    construction of 19–20, 26; cultural
    13, 19–20, 29–30; and eating
    disorders 16; and eating properly
    28–9; exterior 20–1, 21–3; and
    fatness 22–3; and food 30; and food
    cultures 29–30; health 26–7; and
    individualism 30; life cycle 23–4;
    self 26; social 13, 19, 27; and
    status 22; and thinness 21–2
illness: and humoral balance 9–13;
    humoral theory 8–9
immunisation 65
imports 94–5, 98
income 34, 64
India 93
individual subjectivity, emergence of
    10–1
individualism, and identity 30
industrialisation 48–9, 77–8, 82
infants, nutrition wisdom 14–5
inner cleanliness 29
interiority of self 11

Irish diaspora 89
Irish potato famine 89
Islam 66

Japan 24
John, King 62
Judaism, dietary laws 63
justice 5; food 87–99; and food
    quality 95–6; and food
    sovereignty 97–8; and food
    technology 93–4; and human
    disaster 90–2; human rights
    89–90; re-establishing 96–7

kitchen gardens 43, 57–8
KPN fertiliser 76

landfill 79
Lang, T. 48
legislation: food supply 61–3, 70–1,
    71; health 66
Leibig, Justus von 76
Lent 66
Lévi-Strauss, Claude 16–7, 18
life: food and 10; food as 12–3
life cycle 23–4
life-skills classes 37
lifestyle correction campaigns 69
lifestyle diseases 65–6
living standards 25–6, 34, 35–6,
    64–5
local food cultures 5
locavore, the 42

mad cow disease 62
Malthus, Thomas 75–6, 90
Maori, the 74–5
Marie Antoinette 89
market segmentation 34–5
marketing 49–50, 50–1, 58, 92
meat industry 95–6
medicine: early 6; humoral theory
    9–13
Menzel, Peter 91
methane 79
Mexico 78

Middle Ages 63
Middle East 74
migration 30, 85, 90–1
milk 15
Moa, the 75
moderation 23, 28, 68
modernity 41
molecular biology 7
Monteiro, Carlos 53
moral character 6, 11
Murcott, Anne 16
Murray Darling Basin drought 80
mutton flaps 96

Nader, Ralph 82
National Food Plan (NFP),
    Australia 73
national security 39–41
Nauru 22
neo-liberalism 69
New Zealand 71, 75, 95–6
Nigeria 22
nutrients 7
nutrition 7
nutrition wisdom 14–5
nutritional sciences 7, 38–9

Obama, Michelle 43
obesity 22–3; childhood 65;
    epidemic 53, 69, 96
ocean environment, impact on 80–2
oil 77
oppression 16
Orbach, Susie 16
Order of Things, The (Foucault) 10–1
outcropping 84
outsourcing 2
overconsumption 58
overfeeding 22–3
overfishing 81
overproduction 49, 94–5

Pacific Islands 96
palatability 54–5
Papua New Guinea 45–6, 47, 56
Peasants' Way, the 98

pecuniary needs 38–9
pester power 35
pesticides 48, 77–8, 79, 84
physiological needs 39
physiology 7, 11
Planet Obesity (Swinburn and Egger)
    69
pleasure 49–50; management of 28
politics 1, 4; *see also* food politics
Politics of Provision, The (Bohstedt)
    88–9
population displacement 30, 85, 90–1
population growth 90;
    environmental impact 75, 75–6
post-swallowing cultures 13, 20
poverty 16
power 22; in the family 34, 36
pre-prepared foods 37; reliance on 41
preservatives 48
pressure groups 83
pre-swallowing cultures 13, 19–20
price wars 51–2
prices 23; and *Big Food* 51, 51–2;
    decrease in 64; drought and
    79–80; feul 77; fresh food 51, 56;
    and overproduction 94–5;
    ultra-processed foods 55
processed culinary ingredients 53
processing 48, 61–2
production inputs 48
production monopolies 52
proper eating 39
proper meals 37
provenance 43, 46, 92, 98
psychological needs, satisfying 18
psychological wellbeing 8
psycho-social-cultural perspectives 13
psycho-somatic wellbeing 10
public health law 61
purchasing power 51
Pure Food Act (UK 1860) 61
purity 29

Ramadan 66
rationality 29; and moderation 28
rationing 40

refrigeration 76
refugee camps 91
regulation 32, 60–71; of affluence
  65–8; ancient Greek 67–8;
  cultural 63–4; definition 4; dietry
  laws 63–4, 66–7; food supply
  61–3; legislation 61–3, 70–1, 71;
  re-establishment of 69–70;
  restraint 66–7, 68–9;
  self-regulation 60, 66–8, 71;
  self-regulation of appetite 64–5; of
  sexual activities 67
relationship with 1–2
religion 28–9, 63–4, 66–7
Renaissance, the 10–2
replenishment processes 21
restraint 64–5, 66–7, 68–9
retail sector 51, 57
rioting 88–9
Ritzler, George 49
role 1–2
Rome 10
Roundup 83
Roundup Ready plants 83
Rowntree, Seebohm 16
ruminant animals, greenhouse gas
  emissions 79

salmon 81–2
salt 55
same-sex relationships 67
Samoa 96
Santich, Barbara 12
Scandinavia 81
schools, garden schemes 57–8
Second World War 36, 40, 41, 48
seed sales 97
self, and humoral theory 11
self identity 26
self-control 23
self-denial 66–7
self-fulfilment 49–50
self-reflection 69
self-regulation 60, 64–5, 66–8, 71
self-sufficiency 46
sexual activities, regulation of 67

sheep, greenhouse gas emissions 79
shopping 54
Silent Spring (Carson) 78, 82
Simpson, Wallace, Duchess of
  Windsor 22
social contagion 27
social development 4
social identity 4, 13, 19, 27
social networks 27
social roles 26
social status 22, 23, 27
soil depletion 4
soil management 76
Southern Ocean, the 81
spiritual significance 28–9
standards of living 25–6, 34, 35–6,
  64–5
Stanley, Ryan 23
starvation 21
status 22, 23, 27
Stephanie Alexander Kitchen
  Garden, Melbourne 43
stockpiling 49
sugar 55
Sumerians, the 74
Sumo wrestlers 22
sumptuary laws 63–4
supermarkets 4, 42, 51, 51–2, 57,
  92, 97
survival 88
sustainability 73, 74, 77, 82, 84, 95
Swinburn, Boyd 69
symbolic capital 27

Tahiti 22
Tait, Gordon 16
taxation 70–1
television 58
temperament 8; humoral
  explanations 9
thinness 21–2
trade, and food justice 94–5
traditional diets, and aging 24
traditional lifestyles 65
transport 79; and fuel prices 77
travel 1

tuna 81
turkey tails 96

ultra-processed foods: children and
55; definition 53; growth 53–5;
health impacts 53–6; marketing
54, 55; and the obesity epidemic
53; palatability 54–5; price 55;
sales 53
understanding 13
United States of America: biofuel
production 95; droughts 95;
household expenditure 23; meat
industry 96; nutritional sciences in
38–9
Universal Declaration of Human
Rights 89–90
unprocessed foods 53
urban food gardens 43
urbanisation 47–8, 56

vegetables 55
vertical integration 52
Via Campestina movement 98
vulnerability 40

waste 50, 68–9, 84
Waste and Resources Action
Programme (WRAP) 68–9
waste disposal 79
waste in vain 84
water 7; availability 91;
rationing 80
wealth, display of 25
weather: climate change 4,
78–80, 85; extreme events
79–80
wellbeing 8, 10
wheat production 76
wildlife, extinctions 75
willpower 23
Wolf, Naomi 16
womanhood 16
women 4; employment 40–1, 53–4;
liberation 56
work–life balance 53–4
World Food Programme 91
World Health Organisation 55
World Trade Organisation 96

you are what you eat 19